GET YOUR TEAM ON BOARD

GROWING YOUR DENTAL BUSINESS

Market Yourself Effectively
and Accelerate Your Results

PENNY REED

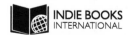

INDIE BOOKS
INTERNATIONAL

ISBN: 1-941870-22-8
ISBN 13: 978-1-941870-22-8
Library of Congress Control Number: 2015936216

Designed by Joni McPherson, mcphersongraphics.com

INDIE BOOKS INTERNATIONAL, LLC
2424 VISTA WAY, SUITE 316
OCEANSIDE, CA 92054
www.indiebooksintl.com

FOR BROOKE AND SAVANAH

*Don't ever let anyone tell you that you aren't
capable of doing whatever you set your mind
to do. If you want it, set a goal and go for it.
You can do it. I believe in you and I love you.*

TABLE OF CONTENTS

Section I

MANAGE TO GROW

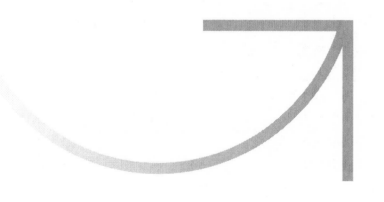

CHAPTER 1

The Evolving Role of the Dentist in Their Practice

The business of dentistry is changing. With every new advance in technology and efficiency it seems there is more that must be monitored and managed to be profitable. Many years ago, dentists had little technology to manage, less competition, fewer out of network concerns, smaller offices, and fewer team members. Now in the world of instant communication, online reputations and comparisons, more competition, higher volume, and lower profit margins a successful and profitable practice requires more management tools to grow.

Many practice owners have a practice administrator or business manager, which is an awesome and exciting addition to the dental team. While the day-to-day operations may be handled by this manager, it is imperative that you—as the business owner—master your roles so that you are guiding the vision and direction of what is likely the greatest investment of finances and time in your career.

A dental business owner has roles that are quite different from a dentist. A dental business owner may be a practicing dentist, but in more recent trends, not every dentist is, or will become, an owner.

Your role can be broken down into three segments: owner/CEO, leader, and coach. The owner/CEO role deals with the concepts we will cover in this book, which are the business benchmarks, systems, and strategies to grow the practice. These concepts are at the core of building and managing a profitable practice. The other segments of leadership and coaching pertain to the qualities and habits the dental business owner must have and must coach their team toward.

You may wonder why it is important for you, as the dental business owner, to worry about such things if you have a business or office manager. If you are an owner who is practicing dentistry, your management skill, leadership, and coaching abilities matter. Why? Because the team will follow your leadership, and the office manager can only manage to the level that you empower them.

In this book you will learn what you need to know to manage the primary components, as well as continue to grow the practice. If I can convey only one message to you as you begin this study and journey, it is this:

It takes time to grow your business.

It isn't a set of quick bells, whistles, and recipes that you can simply toss to your team. You must be deliberate and intentional and keep at it. This starts with you and your understanding and willingness to participate in the "business" of your practice. You must know it, believe it, and live it so you can delegate it. Even then, you need to know where to keep your finger placed so you are adequately tuned in to the pulse of your business. Its performance will speak to you. You need to be sure you are listening and can understand what the messages mean.

Being deliberate and intentional requires investing your time, outside of patient contact time, to exercise your business owner muscles. Just like patients' appointments are scheduled in your management software, your time to work on the business must be placed on your schedule. How much time? Four hours per month is a great place to start. Some may not need this much and others, who aren't at all familiar with their numbers, may need more. The ideal would be one hour per week.

This is a focused hour, with no interruptions. It's easiest to have this time at the office, or it can be done from a home office if you have remote access or have your reports with you. This hour is "Elvis has left the building" time. Let your team know not to interrupt you during this time unless there is a true emergency, and that you will follow up with them when you have completed reviewing the practice stats. Set yourself up for success; don't check e-mail, take phone calls, or surf the Internet. If you don't put this framework around this time, it will be filled with distractions, and you will feel like you are spending tons of time "on" the business but getting nowhere.

Ready? If you are the type of reader that rarely finishes a book, in the next chapter I will give you an overview of how to grow your dental business, right up front. The rest of the book will teach you, step-by-step, how to get those results. I encourage you to read the entire book and get actively involved. You may want to grab a notebook, journal, or iPad to take notes as you read along to create action plans. Go ahead and schedule that administrative time each week now. Now you have already accomplished something to improve your business before we even really get started.

CHAPTER 2

Five Keys to Growing Your Dental Business

I f you've been in practice for any length of time, you've likely read dozens, if not hundreds, of articles on how to grow your practice. The purpose of this book is to direct your focus to the five areas that drive growth in your business and how your role as a business owner, leader, and coach influence these key areas.

Every aspect of growing your dental business falls under one of these strategies:

1. Increase New Patients

2. Increase Active Patients

3. Increase Hygiene Membership

4. Increase Case Acceptance

5. Increase Efficiency

Let's go ahead and put pen to paper and look at how small amounts of growth in each area can have a great impact on your dental business.

1. Increase New Patients by 10 Percent

A thriving dental practice should have a minimum of twenty-five New Patients (comprehensive exams) per full-time doctor per month.

If the value of a new patient is $2,000, and we increase 10 percent, or three New Patients per month, your revenue would increase like this:

3 Additional New Patients per month at

$2,000 per New Patient =

$6,000 per month in additional Production

$72,000 Annual Production increase

2. Increase Active Patients by 10 Percent

Increasing active patients means, not only adding new patients, but also ensuring the total active patient base is growing and not shrinking. In a practice with 2000 Active Patients, (an Active Patient is a patient who has been in to the office in the last twenty-four months), an increase in 10 percent would translate to increased revenue.

If the last 24 months Production = **$2,400,000**

# of patient visits over last 24 months = **12,000**

32 patients per day, 4 days per week

50 weeks per year

Average value per patient visit **$200**

10 percent increase = **200** more active patients

$200 value per visit X **200** additional active patients =

$40,000 Annual Production Increase

3. Increase Hygiene Membership 10 Percent

You can have more patients in the practice see the hygienist regularly to increase revenue and overall dental health.

Active Patients: **2000**

Potential Recare Appointments Needed =

2000 Active Patients X **2** or **4000** Recare Appointments

If a practice conducts 1600 periodic evaluations per year, they have 40 percent Recare Effectiveness (1600 Periodic

Evals divided by 4000 potential is 40 percent Recare Effectiveness)

To increase Hygiene Membership by 10 percent (to 50 percent) – 2000 periodic evaluations are needed. We can break those numbers down even further:

An increase of **400** recall visits annually

An increase of **33** recall visits monthly: **$149** – Periodic eval, Avg Adult/Child Prophy, ½ of the Two-Bitewing fee – no FMX (full mouth x-ray), Panorex or Flouride

Additional Monthly Production: **$4967**

$59,600 Increased Annual Production

4. Increase Case Acceptance by 5 Percent

If the patient visit value is $200, and we increase it by 5 percent, we raise the value by $10 per patient visit for a total of $210 per patient visit average.

That change produces an additional income of $10 per visit at 6144 visits per year.

The monthly increase would be $5,120, with a $61,440 Annual Increase.

5. Maximize Efficiency of Provider Time by 10 Percent

In an eight hour day, this would mean streamlining systems to allow almost an additional hour of primary provider time (doctor or hygienist).

We will focus on freeing up thirty minutes (three ten-minute units) of primary time in operative and the same amount for hygiene.

> **200** Patient contact days (**4** days per week, **50** weeks per year)
>
> **$1,200,000** Gross Revenue
>
> **$5970** Production Per Day
>
> **$746** Production Per Hour
>
> If OP produces **65** percent: **$485** per hour
>
> If HYG produces **35** percent : **$261** per hour

If we become 10 percent more efficient, this is thirty minutes opened up (or three units on a ten-minute schedule) per department's schedule, per day.

> **$242.54** Operative Time Added Per Day
>
> **$130.60** Hygiene Time Added Per Day
>
> **$6,250** in Time Efficiency Added Monthly
>
> **$75,000** Efficiency Added Annually

Looking at all these small increases together from the
Five Keys:

$1,200,000 Practice

$72,000 – Increased New Patients

$40,000 – Increased Active Patients

$59,600 – Increased Hygiene Membership

$61,440 – Increased Case Acceptance

$75,000 – Increased Efficiency

$308,040 Potential Growth Opportunity

25 percent increase overall

See the potential? We'll begin our journey on how to
grow your dental business with these five keys and the
importance of your roles as an entrepreneur, leader, and
coach in making these a reality to make and keep your
practice more profitable. The purpose of this book is to
direct your focus to the five areas that drive growth in
your business, which fall into three broader categories:
Marketing, Engagement, and Organization. But first,
let's take some time to understand your financial and
tracking tools.

Section II

FINANCIAL TOOLS

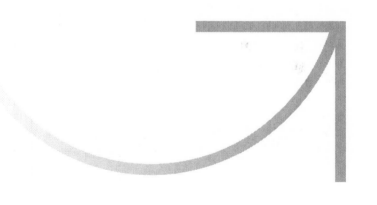

CHAPTER 3

The Importance of Knowing Your Numbers

If you are like many dentists in practice, you went to dental school to improve smiles and help people. Running a business was probably not one of your primary objectives. Yet, here you are with your own practice or even multiple locations. The investment in your dental degree and dental business are likely the most significant investments you will ever make. You need to ensure that you are getting a sound return on that investment.

How do you know if you are making money? To be successful, you must understand what your current financials mean and track them regularly. You may be thinking, "Hey, I already know I need to make more money; I want to start with that part." It's tempting, I know. But, think of the profitability of your practice as a map. When you look up a location on a map and try to make a plan to get to a destination, you must know your current location. This is the best way to determine how you are going to get where you want to go.

It's not only important to know what you are tracking, but also the best way to track the numbers and what they really mean. You might be thinking, "Whoa, that's why I have an office manager." My hope is that you will trust me and listen to my advice based on more than twenty years of experience. Having a qualified office manager can be a vital component to growing and managing your business. Yet, if the office manager is the only one who knows your numbers, you are not only prime material for embezzlement, you are going to be in for a rollercoaster ride when your office manager leaves.

As the owner, you should have a better handle on your numbers than anyone else in the business. Yes, your office manager should know them too. You should share some numbers with your team. The more educated your team is about how to make and keep the business healthy, the more accountable and vested they will be in your practice.

In the following chapters we will look at:

- The numbers you should be tracking

- How to track them

- How often to track them

- What to look for

The Importance of the Income Statement

Let's start with your income statement (or sometimes called profit and loss report). Hopefully you use QuickBooks or a similar bookkeeping software—it is likely the system you use to write checks and/or do payroll. I highly recommend you utilize it in your office for paying bills and recording deposits. Most accountants can interface with QuickBooks and you can send them your numbers each month with a click of a button. Even if you use an internal or external bookkeeper to write your checks, the benefit of QuickBooks is real-time tracking of your income and expenses. Not necessarily for tax purposes, but to be able to know weekly and monthly how much has been deposited and spent.

I work with many dentists who have a team member pay bills for them. That is fine to let this work be done by them; however, never, ever allow an office manager or bookkeeper to have authorization to sign your checks. What are the exceptions? The person is a spouse of an owner or you have a group practice and have your own CFO. Even then, you should carefully monitor the income and expense reports. It's usually the people you would never imagine stealing from you who are the first to do it.

If you have a single office or smaller group of practices, I strongly recommend you take a QuickBooks class. I am not asking you to balance your checkbook or figure out your own taxes. You still need an accountant and it's very likely you may also want a bookkeeper. But don't be in the dark. You will never regret having the knowledge of how the program works and how to run the reports. This way, if you do have a new office manager come on board, you are not at the mercy of his or her skill level to be able to get the information you need.

Similarly, one of my successful former clients told me that when he first came into his current practice almost twenty years ago, the senior dentist had him filing his own dental claims by hand. Why? Because the senior dentist knew how important it would be that this young dentist know what was going on the claims. When was the last time you looked at a blank dental claim form? As an owner, it is crucial that you understand all the aspects of the practice's business dealings.

Be sure to review your Income Statement or Profit and Loss Report monthly. You want to view it on a cash basis. There are many items that may look like an expense for tax purposes but aren't actually things you are paying for. You only want to view monies coming in and going out.

In most cases, you will have only one income account for your practice. This is the easiest part to set up. The trickiest part is being sure your expense accounts are setup correctly. Your expenses will fall into two broad categories:

1. **Fixed Expenses** – With a fixed expense, the bill is the same amount each month, no matter how many days you see patients or whether or not the office is open or closed.

    Examples of fixed expenses are:

    - Rent/Note on the office: 3.5 percent

    - Marketing and Advertising: 2 to 5 percent

    - Equipment: 2 percent

    - Telephone and Utilities: 1.75 percent

    - Consulting and CE Expense: 2.5 percent

    In a general practice, your fixed expenses should be no more than 22 percent.

2. **Variable Expenses** – Here variable expenses vary depending on factors such as how many days you work, how many people are working, how many dental supplies you use, etc. In other words, variable expenses increase and decrease based upon the volume in the practice and the hours it is open.

Examples of variable expense benchmarks in a general practice are:

- Dental Office Staff Salaries: 20-22 percent

- Employee Payroll Taxes and Benefits: 3 percent

- Dental Supplies: 5 percent

- Office Supplies: 2 percent

- Dental Lab (internal and external): 11 percent

In a general practice, variable expenses should be no more than 43 percent of collections.

Owners' salaries may be listed as an expense, but they are actually profit to the owner. You want your practice overhead to be no more than 65 percent. You are shooting for a 35 percent profit to owners, minimum. We have clients with overhead figures as low as 45 percent. The important thing is to work toward getting your bottom line in shape and keeping it that way.

You should run your profit and loss report monthly, by the tenth of the month. You want to be sure you use the option to show each item as an expense of collections. Be sure to set up your report so that you can see the previous month's stats (the month that just ended), the year-to-date stats, and both the previous year's stats for the same month and same time period year-to-date.

You must plan to spend about thirty minutes per month reviewing these figures to be sure you understand where your money is going. You work too hard to let it fly out the door.

Knowing Your Numbers – Knowing What to Track in Your Practice Management Software (PMS)

We live in an exciting time of technology in dentistry. I still remember, in my early consulting days, working with clients who did all of their billing and claims manually. The office manager used a ledger book or pegboard system to track numbers and manage accounts receivable. All dental claims were done by hand. Needless to say, it wasn't very efficient.

Now we have some very advanced practice management software, or PMS, systems. For some reason, these software programs are intimidating to some dentists, and they rely solely on their teams to enter data and pull reports. This is becoming less common, yet if you must ask a team member to run a report for you because you don't know how, it's time to invest in some training on how to utilize your software. The good news is that the larger PMS companies have great online tutorials and videos. One of my favorite shortcuts to looking something up in a client office is to have a pdf version of their software manual. This way I can quickly pull up references to the data I wish to track.

Here are some useful statistics to track in order to help you understand the business from several different perspectives.

Collections: This is one of the most, if not the most, critical statistic to track. Collections refers to the amount the practice has been paid for procedures rendered. Usually Collections are broken down into two categories:

- **Gross Collection** is the total dollars received into the practice, before any credits or refunds.

- **Net Collection** is the net amount of money received into the practice after any refunds or adjustments.

Production: The best "business" term for Production is items sold and delivered. This is the amount the patient is charged for the service or product. Production is also broken down into two categories:

- **Gross Production** is the amount charged for a procedure, at the practice's full fee, before any discounts or adjustments.

- **Net Production** is the net amount charged for the procedure, after discounts or PPO adjustments.

The easiest way to describe Net Production is the amount that is charged to the patient that is actually collectible.

Many practices focus solely on Gross Production and build their business plan around that figure. A better figure to look at as far as goal setting is Net Production. You can only get paid for the dollar amount that is collectible. So when we get to the chapter on Smart Dental Scheduling, we will mainly speak in terms of scheduling to a Net Production goal. This has a greater impact on practices that offer discounts and participate in PPO plans.

Production by Department or Income Center: In general, pediatric, and periodontal practices, Production is usually tracked by departments as well as providers.

- **Hygiene Department:** Hygiene production is defined as production that takes place in the hygiene department. This includes, but is not limited to, exams, x-rays, prophylaxis, sealants, periodontal treatment, and fluoride. At this point, only a dentist can charge for an exam and x-rays are not billable until they have been interpreted by the dentist. Therefore, many practices show the production for the exams and x-rays done in hygiene as doctor production. This is perfectly acceptable. It is also important to look at the actual production (total) that takes place in the Hygiene Department, meaning any production that takes place in a hygiene room as hygiene production. Many offices work around this by having two different provider numbers in the PMS for each dentist. What should the hygiene department produce? If exams and x-rays are included in the hygiene production, hygiene should produce 35 to 40 percent of practice production. If exams and x-rays are credited to the dentists, hygiene should produce 25 to 35 percent of the practice production.

- **Operative Department:** Operative production is defined as production that takes place in the operative department. This usually includes fillings, crowns, bridges, dentures, partials, implants, endodontics, extractions, etc.

- **Orthodontics Department:** In a general or pediatric dental practice that has an orthodontist on staff or performs orthodontics, it's a great idea to track these procedures to see the percentage of overall production that comes from orthodontic procedures. It allows you to focus on the growth of this revenue stream when you break it out as an income center.

- **Aesthetics Department:** In some states, dentists are allowed to perform cosmetic procedures that were not traditionally provided in a dental practice.

Botox, dermal fillers, and other facial aesthetics are an income center being added to many practices across the United States. The rules on whether a dentist can perform these procedures are state specific. Before you add rooms, chairs, equipment, supplies, and staffing to add these facial aesthetic procedures to your practice, be sure to check with your dental board and get their stance on it in writing. If you practice in a state where these services can be conducted in your office, you will also want to track these statistics separately so you can see if providing them more than covers your cost to provide them.

Production by Provider: Your PMS also tracks production by provider, based upon the procedures that are entered. These figures are important for tracking individual provider (doctor or hygienist) productivity. This is especially important to know when comparing actual production to daily goals by provider or if you have hygienists on commission and/or associate or partner dentists who are compensated based on production. It's also important when calculating commission based on collections. The work must be produced before the income can be collected.

Report of Production by Procedure (aka Procedure Analysis): This report has a gold mine of information on it. Not only can you track how many of each procedure is being conducted, but also the production from those procedures. In addition, this report can be sorted by provider so you may see how many of a certain procedure were done by doctor or hygienist. For example, if you have more than two doctors, and you want to determine how many D0150 Comprehensive exams each doctor has done for a time period, this is the report. The data from the Production by Procedure report is valuable not only in comparing provider productivity, but it is also useful for computing the number of patients active in hygiene as well as case acceptance. We will touch more on those points in their respective chapters.

Accounts Receivable and Outstanding Insurance: Accounts Receivable is the amount of money owed to the practice, by insurance and patients, for treatment that has already been rendered. A healthy Accounts Receivable amount should be no greater than one times the average monthly Net Production. In other words, if a practice averages $150,000 per month in Net Production, there should be no greater than $150,000 in Accounts Receivable. The exception is Orthodontic practices, which tend to carry greater Accounts Receivable due to the nature of the treatment. In those cases the patients on payment plans are much greater and the practice has the advantage of spreading the treatment out over many months.

The key to keeping the Accounts Receivable manageable is to work it consistently each day. The benchmarks should be:

- Current (less than 30 days old) – 66 percent

- 30 to 60 days old – 10 to 13 percent

- 60 to 90 days old – 10 to 13 percent

- Over 90 days old – no greater than 8 percent

One of the key strategies for effectively managing Accounts Receivable is to offer outside financing sources. Some of these allow the patient to spread their payments over twelve to eighteen months with no interest. Other options are lower payments over a longer period of time at a specified rate of interest.

Outstanding Insurance is a component within the Accounts Receivable that is owed, or estimated to be owed, by the dental benefits company. The portion of Accounts Receivable that will be segmented by Outstanding Insurance varies depending on the number of patients in the practice with dental benefits. If a practice's patient base is primarily composed of fee-for-service patients, the Outstanding Insurance may only make up 15 to 20 percent of the Accounts Receivable. If a practice is more heavily composed of patients with dental benefits, the Outstanding

Insurance may be more in the range of 60 to 70 percent of the Accounts Receivable.

Keys to keeping insurance reimbursement simple are to file claims electronically, including the attachments. In addition, file claims daily. Accurate treatment notes make the job of the administrative team easier as the clinical record should contain any information that might be needed in a narrative. Also, be sure to include supporting documentation, x-rays, photos, initial placement or replacement, periodontal charting, etc., with the claim.

Days and Hours Worked: As we delve deeper into knowing your numbers, you will find it vital to know not only how many hours the practice was open and treating patients, but also how many days and hours each provider worked each month. While some PMS track this for you, if you use an integrated time-clock, this is an item that is usually tracked with a spreadsheet or manually on paper. Here is how I recommend you track days and hours worked by provider:

In a practice with one doctor and one hygienist, if both of them work on a day, that is:

1 Day for the Practice

1 Doctor Day

1 Hygiene Day

In a practice with one doctor and two hygienists, if all three of them work on a day that is:

1 Day for the Practice

1 Doctor Day

2 Hygiene Days

And in a practice with two dentists and three hygienists, if all five of them work on a day that is:

1 Day for the Practice

2 Doctor Days

3 Hygiene Days

In other words, each day that each doctor works is counted as a doctor day and each day that a hygienist works is counted as a hygiene day.

To continue to clarify, in the last example, where we had two dentists and three hygienists, if each dentist worked four days last week, that would be eight doctor days. And if each hygienist worked four days last week, that would be twelve hygiene days. The practice was open Monday through Friday, so that is five practice days.

Tracking the figures this way gives us more flexibility in measuring our productivity, as well as our efficiency. This will make more sense as we calculate value per chair hour and, equally as important, individual provider productivity by day and by hour.

Chair Hour Value and Why It's Important

What is the value of a chair hour in your practice? When I ask this question to most dental business owners, they aren't sure of the answer. Yet, this is one of the most important stats in the practice. It's one of the most vital, yet it's not the simplest to calculate.

Chair hour value is calculated by reviewing the following (figures below are referenced for the previous twelve months):

1. Number of hours the office is open to see patients.

2. Number of chairs utilized in the practice for patient care (total number of chairs, for operative and hygiene if applicable).

3. Practice collections.

4. Practice income statement (showing all expenses by category).

5. Monthly notes payable which aren't reflected on the

income statement. This may include, but is not limited to, practice purchase note and/or equipment note.

First, you will multiply the number of hours the practice is open times the number of chairs utilized for patient care. For example, in a practice open five days per week with five chairs that is closed ten business days per year, the calculation would look like this:

> **50** weeks of patient care per year
>
> **40** hours of patient care per week
>
> **5** chairs utilized for patient care
>
> equals
>
> **10,000** chair hours per year available for
>
> patient care and revenue generation

Next, take the last twelve months collections, and divide it by the number of chair hours the practice had available. In this example we will use 1.5 million in collections.

> **1,500,000** collections divided by **10,000** hours = **$150** per chair hour collections
>
> In a practice with a **98** percent collections ratio, this is **$153** per chair hour production

Now that we know what the practice generated per chair hour, we need to see what the break-even is per chair hour—also known as our cost per chair hour. This is done by taking the overhead dollars from the income statement (again for the last twelve months), as well as annual amounts spent on practice and equipment notes, which most often aren't reflected on the income statement.

In this example, the practice has an overhead (expenses not including doctor's salary) of $900,000. For this calculation, we figure existing or base staff salaries as a fixed cost. The reason is, unless they are on commission or you send them home when the schedule is light, you are spending those dollars on staffing. A little later, we will cover how to factor in adding staffing and the impact it will have on the chair hour cost.

Here is the recommended way to segment these expenses for computing chair hour cost:

Fixed costs (for chair hour cost calculation)
Approximately 40 Percent
Rent or Building Note
Build-out and/or Renovation Note
Equipment Note
Staffing Cost
Payroll Taxes (staff only)
Other Taxes
Legal and Accounting

Professional Dues

Consulting and CE

Travel

Business Insurance

Postage

Utilities, Internet, and Phone

Repairs and Maintenance

Variable Costs – Expenses that increase directly with production – Approximately 20 Percent

Lab

Dental Supplies

Office Supplies

Advertising Expense

Bank and Credit Card Expense

Now that you have your expenses listed and tallied, you can review your overhead per chair hour also known as "break-even per chair hour."

$900,000 expenses for the last 12 months, divided by 10,000 chair hours equals = $90 break-even per chair hour. This means, based upon the days and hours worked as well as chairs utilized, each chair must generate $90 per hour simply to cover overhead.

Why is knowing the break-even per chair hour so important? When evaluating insurance plan participation or adding and/or staffing additional chairs, it's critical to know what the overhead is per chair per hour. This is how you know whether or not you will make money, and how much, for adding additional working space. It's also how you will know whether or not you can afford to participate in certain plans, based upon their reimbursement.

There are many ways that knowing your break-even or cost per chair hour can help you to make decisions. Let's refer back to the practice in our example. Let's say there is a sixth room that is equipped and ready to use, but has not been staffed. You are thinking of adding additional hygiene days to the schedule. Let's say you added three more days of hygiene per week. This would be an additional 1,200 chair hours added per year.

Now let's look at the cost to staff that additional room. Let's say your staff cost will increase $45,000 and your additional costs will be the supplies used to see those additional patients. If the hygiene chair produces $1,200 per day, and supplies run approximately 5 percent, the supplies will run approximately $60 per day. Therefore, the additional overhead annually to book hygiene in the seventh room for three days per week is $54,000.

How does that change the numbers? We've added 1,200 chair hours for a total of 11,200 chair hours annually. And now our overhead (if we take the last twelve months' figures) would be $954,000. Therefore our new break-even per chair hour is $85.18.

Remember, knowledge is power, and the more you know about your practice statistics, the better decisions you will make. Before you add another team member, operatory, or an associate, be sure you know these numbers so you can project the financial impact it will have on your bottom line.

CHAPTER 4

Goal Setting and Team Bonuses

You may wonder why these two are paired together in the same chapter. It's because you cannot have a bonus system that is a win-win for the doctor and team without being sure the practice goals support generating enough revenue to allow for team bonuses. Bonuses for the team are a huge boost for morale and productivity, unless the system is setup without advanced planning and the rules have to be changed and the bonus is reduced or taken away.

Here is a step-by-step approach to setting up a bonus system that gives incentive to the team, and quite a nice one when the numbers are there, and also protects the owner.

First, you must look at the income statement. On an annual basis, add together both fixed and variable costs, along with practice notes. Next add in your owner's income goal (for all owners), and this gives you your bare minimum goal so that all of the practice bills are paid and the owners are paid. As a note, owners should be paid a minimum of 35 percent of the practice collections before taxes (this would be divided by all owners).

Next, let's begin with the goal setting process. In the business of dentistry, our facility and equipment costs are significant and can run upwards of 15 to 20 percent. In many cases we are able to pay off equipment notes and building notes. Yet the one ongoing expense, which usually exceeds the facility expense, is staffing. We cannot serve our patients well without our team. In most practices, staff salaries will be the greatest expenditure, and rightly so. A great team will make or break a practice.

In general dentistry, staff salaries should be close to 20 percent of collections. The same is true for most periodontal practices. Other specialties such as endodontics, oral surgery, orthodontics, and pediatric offices may have lower staff salaries, in the range of 15 to 18 percent. We'll use the general practice statistic of 20 percent to explain the process.

Let's look at an example: Remember the goal is to keep staff salaries at 20 percent of collections (or less) without exceeding that percentage when paying out bonuses. Therefore if gross staff salaries are 20 percent of collections, and the goal is to keep that at that percentage, we will multiply staff salaries by five (since five is the reciprocal of 20 to 100 percent, or in other words, five is the number we must multiply times 20 percent to see what 100 percent will be). To keep things simple, let's say that gross staff salaries are $20,000 per month. Five times $20,000 equals a base desired break-even collections goal of $100,000 per month, before there is money available for bonuses.

In most cases, this figure, staff salaries time five, is greater than your bare minimum goal that you calculated at the beginning of this section (fixed and variable overhead, plus practice notes and desired owner income). If not, you will want to use the bare minimum goal as your collections before bonus.

Let's continue along with the example where our desired break-even collections goal is $100,000. In this scenario, we will bonus the team 20 percent of collections, over the base goal, on a three month rolling average. There are several reasons for using a three month average:

1. It prevents the practice from paying bonuses on this month's figures when last month's collections alone might not have been enough to pay the practice overhead.

2. If the practice experiences a low collections month this month, but had great collections the prior two

months, the team may still be eligible for some sort of bonus.

3. It prevents the temptation, if the team sees they aren't going to hit goal this month, of deciding this month isn't worth trying to salvage and encouraging patients to schedule next month.

So the formula looks like this:

> Last three months average collections – Last three months average staff salaries x five
> = the dollar amount over break-even.
>
> Next, take the dollar amount over break-even and multiply times 20 percent.
>
> This gives you the amount available for team bonuses for that month, referred to as the bonus pool.
>
> Divide the bonus pool by the number of team members
>
> And this gives you the amount of bonus per team member.

Here's an example using the $100,000 break-even collections figure to compute the bonus for March:

Collections

January $115,000

February $110,000

March $117,000

Total is $342,000 and three month average is $114,000

Staff Salaries x Five (Break-even Goal)

January $102,000

February $98,000

March $100,000

Total is $300,000 and the three month average is $100,000

Last three month's average collections $114,000 minus last three months Staff salaries x five, $100,000 gives $14,000 over break-even.

Twenty percent of the amount over break-even goes to staff, which is $2,800. If there are six team members, this would be a bonus of $466 per team member for March.

What affects the bonus? The primary factors to impact the amount needed for bonus when using this bonus method are:

- Increases or decreases in number of staff

- Raises given to staff

- Increase or decrease in number of work-days during the month

- Number of pay periods in a month

Why is it so important to base the bonus on collections, not production? This goes back to making the bonus a win-win for the doctors and team. We must produce the work before we can collect it. And we can't pay a bonus out of production. Basing the formula on collections gives the team a vested interest in being sure that appropriate financial agreements are made with patients before the work has begun.

You may wonder why this formula works so well. First, I must emphasize, there is no perfect bonus formula. Yet this one works best because it is a team effort and there is no disputing who gets credit for what. It takes every department to handle a patient from their initial phone call until their work is completed and their account is paid in full.

Before sitting down with the team to ask them what sort of bonus they want to shoot for, we sit down with the doctors and leadership team to be sure they understand the numbers. Next we involve the team and ask them what amount of bonus they want to shoot for each month, reminding them that this is a gross amount, and it will be taxed just like their other wages. The beauty of allowing the team to choose the bonus they want to shoot for is it gives them ownership and builds in accountability.

Let's say the team chooses to shoot for a $700 bonus per individual each month. (Please note, in these examples, the dollars have been rounded.) We must work backwards to compute the goal.

$700 bonus times six team members equals a bonus pool of $4200 which must be multiplied times five to compute the amount over break-even that is needed.

This means we need $21,000 over our break-even goal of $100,000, or $121,000 in collections per month.

Next, take the target collections goal of $121,000 and divide it by the practice collections percentage, to see what the production goal should be. If the practice collections percentage is 98 percent then you would take $121,000 and divide it by 98 percent giving you a net production goal of $123,470.

If the practice sees patients four days per week, this gives approximately sixteen work-days per month. The production goal of $123,470 divided by 16 days is $7,717 per day.

In a general practice, the hygiene department should produce from 35 to 40 percent of the practice production. In this example we will allocate 65 percent to operative and 35 percent to hygiene.

The operative department goal would be $7,717 times 65 percent or $5,016 per day. If the doctor works out of two rooms, this would be $2,508 per chair per day. If the practice sees patients eight hours per day, this would be $314 per chair per hour.

This means the hygiene department goal is $7,717 times 35 percent or $2,701 per day. If there are two hygiene chairs, this is a goal of $1,351 per hygiene chair per day and $169 per chair per hour.

Now we have clarity about what is needed to hit our target bonus goal of $700 per team member, which also exceeds our practice goals based on overhead, notes payable, and doctor's desired income.

Intentional planning and scheduling are keys to reaching the practice goals. If we have time scheduled out of the office for vacation or CE, we may need to make up a day here and there to be sure we don't drop too far below our desired number of work-days each month.

It is ideal to have at least one planning session per year with your team. Bring your practice figures, a large calendar, dates that the office will be closed during holidays and vacations, and begin to map out your schedule. You will also want to review your goals for training and delegation to ensure your team is doing all they can legally and ethically in regards to assisting with patient treatment. Review your state's practice act once per year to be sure you and your team are aware of changes to procedures that can be delegated. Then template your daily schedule, see the chapter on Smarter Dental Scheduling, to ensure each day is properly configured to support you to reach your goals in all departments.

Setting and monitoring goals and actual figures monthly gives you more chances to make corrections than having only annual goals that are reviewed once per year. If you have a bad month, shake it off and go into the next month with a clean slate and a renewed attitude to work your plan.

CHAPTER 5
Fees and Insurance Participation

A few decades ago you would have heard me say never participate in a preferred provider network (PPO). There have been several factors that have shifted that stance, not only for me, but for thousands of dentists across the country. Twenty years ago, there were fewer dentists participating in the plans, meaning that non-plan providers had little to be concerned with as far as competitors with in-network fees. Now there are more companies offering PPO plans, more employees participating in them, and more aggressive marketing techniques by the insurance companies. Younger dentists came into their practices with hefty school loans and no patients in their chairs, and became PPO providers right off the bat. In addition, there is more transparency in every industry regarding fees. In dentistry, patients now have access through the Internet to one of the largest fee databases in the country, www.fairhealthconsumer.org. A patient can visit FairHealth's consumer cost lookup and view as many as five procedures and find an expected fee for their zip code. It's also very common for national corporate dental chains to post the fees for their most common procedures on their website. What does all of this mean? There is more competition in the marketplace and patients are doing their best to be savvy with their dental dollars.

First, let's acknowledge that no one wants to be paid less than "the going rate" for their services. Also we have to address the myth of the write-off. There has been a thought process in the dental industry that write-off equals money you have lost. This would be 100 percent true if you were choosing whether or not to do something for your full fee in room one or for a reduced fee in room two. The main reason the "write-off equals money you have lost" logic is faulty is that most practices don't have an endless supply of patients in the reception area lined up to do the services at the full fee.

Here is a comparison: Big Smiles airlines charges $500 for a round trip ticket from Dallas to New York City. Their plane holds 100 passengers. Grin and Go airlines charges $425 for their same route from Dallas to New York and their plane also holds 100 passengers. What is the difference between the service on these airlines? Big Smile's flight attendants wear cute business suits and offer a full can of soda to their passengers and a choice of peanuts or pretzels. Grin and Go's flight team wears polo shirts and khaki shorts and offers only a small cup of soda and only has pretzels for their passengers. On the average flight, Big Smiles has thirty open seats while Grin and Go has only ten open seats. Which airline generated more money on their flight? Grin and Go generated an additional $3250 on that trip. Do you think there was a buzz in the Grin and Go board room that they lost $75 per ticket because the "usual" fee of Big Smiles was $500? No way, Grin and Go knows that they made more money and that their price point is a competitive edge that brings them more customers. What's even better is that most of the Grin and Go customers know that they saved $75 on their ticket and told all of their friends.

I chose the airline analogy because this is a highly competitive industry with huge overhead and rising costs. Hopefully you can see the similarities to the business operations of a dental practice. With the shift in our economy over the last several years, insurance plan participation is playing a more significant role. Knowing how to tell if you are making money on a plan is a skill that is paramount to your practice profitability.

If you don't participate in any PPOs, you are likely wondering if you should. The answer to your question can be found by looking at the following metrics. A business decision of that magnitude should not be based on emotions alone. Here are key questions to determine whether or not your practice should participate in plans.

1. **What are the demographics in the area where you practice?** There is truly a difference between a white collar metropolitan area and a blue collar more urban area. Another factor that comes into play is the number of dentists in an area. When it comes down to basics, it is a basic supply and demand lesson in economics. The greater the demand for dentistry is in an area, the easier it is for a dentist to receive their full fee and avoid plan participation. The more saturated an area is with dentists, the lesser the demand.

2. **How many active patients do you have and is that number growing or shrinking?** Many times dentists ask us how many active patients they need. A general practice should have a minimum of 1000 patients that are active in their system. An ideal number is closer to 1500. How do you measure active patients? An active patient is one who has been in your practice for some type of office visit in the past twenty-four months.

Be sure to monitor those patients who leave the practice. The owners should review monthly what patients have requested a transfer of records and why. Be sure to keep stats on the reasons patients are leaving. A practice that loses one or two patients per month to go to a participating provider is in a totally different situation than a practice that loses eight to ten patients per month.

3. **Is the practice being effectively marketed and are the efforts bringing in the desired number of new patients?** A thriving general practice should have approximately twenty-five new patients per month, per full-time dentist. Evaluate how many comprehensive exams you perform each month. If that number is nowhere close to reaching twenty-five, review your marketing efforts. How effective is the team at asking existing patients for referrals? What amount of the practice budget is being spent on marketing? A healthy range for marketing expenses is 3 to 5 percent of practice collections. New patients are the life-blood of any practice.

Remember, your patients with benefits have a social network of friends and family that may or may not have benefits. Yes, patients who are in-network, if they are happy, will refer not only their in-network coworkers, but also anyone they know. Every new patient you see has the potential to refer their inner circle to you. And more new patients leads to more active patients, and more active patients is the goal of any growing practice.

A final aspect to review in a team meeting is how easy you can make it for a patient to join your practice. We have clients who have experienced massive success by offering a one-time complimentary exam and x-rays to their new patients. This removes the barrier of fees over the phone and allows you to have the insurance conversation face to face, after a relationship has been established with the patient.

4. **Is the practice operating efficiently?** If your practice seems to have an abundance of new patients and yet you struggle to be profitable, this could indicate issues with scheduling efficiency and making the most out of delegating to your team. Over the next thirty days, time your procedures. Be sure the assistants keep track of the amount of primary (doctor/hygienist) and secondary time. Acquaint yourself with your practice act and go back through the procedures and count up the time a primary provider spent doing a function that could have been delegated.

5. How much open chair time is available?

Once you have completed the previous efficiency evaluation, you may now evaluate the amount of open time on your schedule. Track it in ten minute units and separate it out by open doctor time and open hygiene time. Few things cost a practice more than open chair time. In most practices, 20 percent of the practice overhead goes toward fixed costs, and those expenses must be paid whether you see 100 or 1000 patients per month. The other major component to overhead is your direct expenses (staff payroll, associate compensation, lab and dental supplies). These direct expenses run about 40 percent in most general practices. Once the basic overhead is met, the cost to see additional patients is about $.40 for every $1.00 produced. If the schedule is managed effectively, increasing volume through plan participation can be very profitable.

6. Is your active patient base growing or shrinking?

This has not been a stat that has been monitored routinely in practice management. By active patient base, I am referring to the number of people who have been in to see you in the last twenty-four months, not the ones who are flagged active in your software system. Once a practice begins to shrink there is nothing to prevent a snowball effect. Patients talk to their coworkers about why they left their non-participating dentist and how happy or unhappy they are with their new provider. Be sure to check your number of active patients, those who have been in during the last twenty-four months, at least once per quarter.

So, maybe your practice already participates in one or more PPOs and at times you wonder if you are making a wise choice or a mistake. It's usually after you receive an insurance EOB—explanation of benefits—that frustrates you. Here are factors to consider when you already participate, and wonder if you should continue to do so:

First, determine how much income each plan contributes to the practice. In order to do this, start with an individual participatory plan. We'll refer to this plan as XYZ. Next, find out how much money did XYZ benefit plan bring into your practice over the past twelve months? This figure will include not only direct payments to the practice by XYZ benefit plan, but also paid to the practice by the patients who have XYZ benefit plan. Once you have this combined total, divide it by the total practice collections to determine what percent of your practice income came from XYZ benefit plan. For example, if XYZ benefit plan paid $100,000 to your practice and patients of XYZ benefit plan paid $200,000 out of pocket, the total value from participating in XYZ plan is $300,000. If the practice income is $1,000,000, then XYZ benefit plan and its customers, your patients, make up 30 percent of the practice income.

The next step is to determine how much appointment time went to the patients with XYZ participatory plan. This can be done through a random manual audit or through your practice management software. Contact your vendor and let them know what you are looking for. If XYZ plan occupied 25 percent of your chair time, but brought you 30 percent of your income, as in the prior computation, you are making money on the plan. If XYZ plan patients occupied 40 percent of your chair time and only brought in 30 percent of your revenue, there is an issue that needs to be addressed.

Are the participatory plans killing your schedule or do you need to schedule smarter?
I cannot emphasize enough that the appropriate templating and managing of the appointment book can make or break practice profitability. Too often we see practices who schedule every restorative procedure for an hour or who schedule by gross production rather than by net production (the net production is what is actually collectible). By utilizing Smarter Dental Scheduling (see efficiency chapter), each day must have an intentional and appropriate mix of procedures. In addition, each and every team member needs to continuously improve their skills and be flexible by welcoming as many patients as

possible to stay today and have treatment done if it can be done given the current day's schedule.

Last, but not least, talk with your patients.
Choose a few patients that you feel you have a good relationship with, who participate in XYZ plan, and ask them how great of an impact plan participation is in them choosing to see you and staying with your practice.

If you decide to stay out or remove yourself from PPO participation, be careful how you address this with your patients. I strongly recommend avoiding comments like, "We just cannot provide quality care, use quality supplies, or work with good dental labs if we participate with insurance plans." Why wouldn't you want to say this? Because one day you may decide to participate (either for the first time or rejoin a plan) and you don't want your patients to think you are now cutting corners on quality.

Here is a suggestion for what to say when they ask why you aren't in network. "Mrs. Jones, we have dozens of patients that have XYZ dental plan, and it's wonderful that you have dental benefits. Over half of our patients have no dental coverage. I wish we could participate, and yet I have seen too many situations where the patient's desired treatment wasn't a covered benefit by the plan, and the lower reimbursement as a PPO provider puts a time pressure on me that in some cases reduces the time I would like to spend with a patient. I value you as a patient and hope that like other patients in the practice, you will find the few dollars difference in the cost of your care to be money well spent."

How you handle plan participation is becoming more and more important as the patient's dollars are squeezed and they work to be savvy by maximizing their plan benefits in the present economy. The dental practices that continue to provide a high level of quality and service while learning to be flexible and effectively utilize their chair time will continue to grow and experience success.

Section III
MARKETING TOOLS

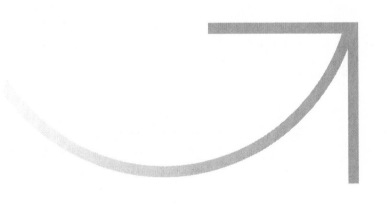

CHAPTER 6

Increasing Your New Patients

What is marketing, and why is it so important? Marketing is the backbone of not only attracting, but also retaining, patients. Marketing is more than advertising. Marketing is the message you deliver. Advertising is simply the medium or vehicle for that message.

As we zone in and focus on the first key of growing your dental business, marketing and attraction move to the forefront. We must do our best to take off our "dental professional" lenses and look at our dental business from the perspective of the patients. What do they want?

- **Quality** – Patients expect a quality product. This means that what they pay for is going to work for them, and they expect it in a clean, sterile environment.

- **Simplicity** – They want their treatment to be easy to understand.

- **Value** – They want to know they have made a smart choice with their dollars.

- **Appreciation** – Patients want to feel appreciated. They have more choices in selecting a dental provider than ever before. They don't want to feel like they are easily replaced.

- **Convenience** – Patients are not only looking for a convenient location, they also want a variety of hours. Now that corporate dentistry is growing and thriving, your competition is offering evening and weekend appointments, and many patients are beginning to depend on those hours so that they don't have to miss work or school.

In understanding why marketing is so important it is vital for you to know how many new patients you need per month in your business. While this book will be beneficial at any level of practice, we are focusing more on those dental businesses who are beyond the initial start-up phase. A growing dental practice needs at least twenty-five new patients per month, per dentist. For the purpose of this chapter, we are defining a new patient as one who has a comprehensive evaluation. We want to effectively monitor the number of patients who move beyond an emergency visit and convert into a true patient of record.

You will want to look in your practice management software and see how many comprehensive exams you are performing each month to see where you are now.

Next, you will want to calculate a measurement we call your "new patient factor." We will refer to this again in the case presentation chapter. What is the "new patient factor"? It is a rule of thumb to measure the value of a new patient in your practice. This value will differ not only from practice to practice but also from doctor to doctor based upon the types of treatment they recommend and perform as well as their ability to sell and gain acceptance of that treatment.

Here is how to calculate your new patient factor:

Average monthly production divided by average monthly comprehensive exams = new patient factor

If a practice has one dentist and averages $80,000 in monthly production and forty comprehensive exams per month, the formula will be as follows:

$80,000 monthly production

divided by

40 comprehensive exams per month

= $2,000 new patient factor

This means the average value a new patient contributes to the practice is $2,000.

And for another scenario, if a solo dental practice averages $120,000 in monthly production and has forty new patients per month, their new patient factor formula will be as follows:

$120,000 monthly production

divided by

40 comprehensive exams per month

= $3,000 new patient factor

It would be a good exercise to calculate the new patient factor in your own office or locations using this formula.

In the example we gave in the introductory chapter, we referred to a goal of 10 percent increase of new patients. In the latter example, a 10 percent increase in new patients, when we average forty per month, is an additional four new patients per month, or one per week. When we focus on the specifics of what we need, it is easier to hit our goals.

In the age of the Internet, digital marketing, and social media, many practices have lost focus on what it takes to attract new patients. I've watched practices spend thousands of dollars per month on a combination of website, Internet pay-per-click ads, and social media packages and receive minimal results. Do you need a website? Absolutely. Is it important that you can be found on the Internet? Of course. Should you have a presence on social media? Definitely. Will these components alone catapult you to your next level marketing goals? Unlikely.

Why? Because marketing has more to do with the message than the vehicle. Yes, you need to be visible, but more importantly, you need to have a strong identity within the practice. Remember, we have to think like a patient. Where do we start?

Booking Visits on the First Call

Why is it so important to make it easy for the patient to join our practice? Because every time a prospective new patient calls, we must change our mindset that we want that new patient scheduled, on the first call. Why? Because in most cases they won't call back if they don't schedule on the first call.

We must remember that the telephone is our initial "connection" with the patient. This is likely one of the most important marketing components you will ever have, and most dental administrators have had little training on how to influence callers to schedule. They are also confused about their purpose on the phone with a prospective new patient. Why? Because many dental business owners and team members don't realize that:

> *The patient must enter your store in order to buy dentistry from you.*

Twenty years ago it was more important to "screen" patients over the telephone to see if they were the right fit for your practice. This is a huge mistake. You don't really know the prospective patient and their needs, wants, and values until you are sitting side-by-side and knee-to-knee with them. Sadly, many practices don't have a new patient issue, they have a telephone issue.

Make It Easy For Patients to Join Your Practice

Two decades ago when I was a dental office manager, business was different. There was less competition, few PPOs, and patients didn't have the luxury of social media to rapidly communicate with their friends.

Now we have more competition and patients who are becoming more savvy with pricing their healthcare. We must have a new mindset that every person who calls and asks questions about joining our practice, treatment, insurance, fees, and hours wants to join our practice. And we need to make it simple for them to do so.

What do I mean? Set your team free to be able to easily schedule new patients into the practice with a zero fee or low fee first visit with necessary x-rays. Offer it to every new patient. Make it easy for your team to invite their friends and family to join your office. Here are a few examples of good introductory offers:

1. Complimentary new patient exam and necessary x-rays (this will be determined by the needs of the prospective new patient). If it's a patient with a specific concern or issue, this will likely be a limited exam and one or two x-rays. If this is a new patient who wants their teeth cleaned, it could be

a comprehensive exam and panorex or full mouth x-rays.

2. Reduced, flat price new patient exam and x-rays. Many offices have had luck with a fee like $10.

Many doctors ask, "What about the production for the exams and x-rays? Can we at least bill their insurance?" The answer is no. If the fee is not billable to the patient, we cannot bill the insurance. This is not only a rule and regulation in the dental practice acts and ADA code of ethics, this is a federal law. I won't spend more of your reading time going into this. If this is a hang-up for you, I am going to coach you to let it go, and focus on watching your new patient numbers, active patients, production, and collections rise.

Some dental teams are resistant to this at first, because they cannot get past not being paid for the initial exam and necessary x-rays. This is an example of stepping over dollars in order to pinch pennies. If your new patient factor is $3,000 per new patient, what would you be willing to spend per new patient in order to acquire them? By the same token, what does it cost you to see a new patient? Let's look at this in the simplest format possible.

If we aren't adding fixed overhead to see new patients (adding chairs), or adding additional team members in order to see new patients, or paying a commission to a team member to see a new patient, and that chair would be empty if the new patients weren't coming in, our additional cost (which is a direct cost) for seeing the new patients is our cost of supplies, which as we've already noted is fairly low. Remember, the offer is for new patients only. They can only get the complimentary exam and x-rays one-time, ever.

A dental office should spend 2 to 5 percent of their collections on advertising and practice promotion. In a practice that has net production of $120,000 per month or $1,440,000 per year, and has a 98 percent collections rate, or $1,411,200 annual collections, the annual advertising budget would be between $28,000 and $70,000 per year. This includes all office promotion: website, signage, business cards, online ads, print ads, phonebook ads, gift cards for patients, in-office drawings, etc.

Needless to say, most thriving practices are spending a significant amount of money to attract and acquire new patients. Yet, too many offices are hung up on getting paid as much as possible for this first visit. Wouldn't it be better to acquire the new patient at zero production than to limit the number of new patients we see?

CHAPTER 7

Think Like A New Patient

Many dental practitioners believe that once an appointment is made, the marketing is over. Quite the contrary. Patients make judgments about your office the minute they turn into the parking lot. What are they seeing?

They begin by looking at the exterior of your building, the condition of your parking lot, your landscaping, and your sign. Patients begin to judge the quality of your dentistry and the health of your business by the visual experience that starts before they even get out of their car.

Next, they walk in and observe. Is the sidewalk clean? What about the reception area? Is it up-to-date? Are the magazines organized? Full or empty? Do you have state-of-the-art amenities like large screen televisions and wireless Internet?

Now the patient observes the administrative area. Does a warm and smiling face promptly greet them? Is the administrative area neat and organized or is there clutter everywhere? Piles of papers (insurance EOBs, invoices, etc.) give the patient a feeling of overall disorganization in the practice. Is there any food present? There should be absolutely no food or drinks (other than possibly a discreetly hidden water bottle) in the administrative area. When the patient observes the dental team with food, coffee, and sodas it gives the practice a look of being too casual, unprofessional, and potentially unclean. Keep those items in the break area.

Next, one of the most important areas in the office is the patient restroom. Even if the team occasionally must use this restroom, remember this is for the patient's convenience. It should be up-to-date in paint and décor. An ongoing air freshening system is a good idea. The restroom should also be monitored multiple times during the day to be sure that it is neat and clean and that the trash is emptied. Your patients spend a good deal of time here, and they make many judgments regarding the practice based upon the look and feel of the restroom.

Before the patient even makes it to the operatory, they usually walk through one or more hallways. We must remember that the hallway is not a storage area for outdated technology or our latest supply delivery. The hallways must be kept neat and clean.

Now for the operatories. Store as many supplies as possible out of view of the patient. We are all aware that dentistry creates anxiety for many patients. Educational brochures are excellent, and if they can be stored outside of the patient view it gives a much more neat and organized feel. Be sure to have televisions, which also work as computer monitors in the operatories as well. This is definitely a patient expectation. Replace the old boxy, tube televisions with flat screens.

> Keep your office up-to-date. Patients will assume
> that your dentistry is only as up-to-date as your
> surroundings.

To illustrate this point, I was talking with a mom recently and she mentioned her child recently got braces. When I asked her who she chose to provide this treatment, she mentioned that she went to several orthodontists for a consultation. She told me that the office she chose appeared to be the most up-to-date. When I asked her how she came to that decision, she said, "You could tell from the reception area that the office was more high tech. There were several flat screen televisions with movies and patient education videos." I thought, wow—that's amazing. It isn't the clinical skill, certificates with accomplishments, or advanced CE. It wasn't the office hours or the price. It was the way she perceived the skill of the orthodontist based upon the appearance/experience in the reception area.

What are other experiences and amenities that patients look for? Much of that will depend on the type of practice you have. Remember, while your practice may see a variety of patients (male, female, various ages, etc.), we are mainly trying to please "Mom." Remember the phrase, "When momma ain't happy, nobody's happy?" Whether a woman is a mom or not, it's usually her decision making that influences others in her life, whether spouse, children, other family members, or friends. Here is a list of questions and concerns mentioned by other women/moms.

- What items are available to "distract" my child or me during dental treatment? Are there televisions in the rooms or are iPods available? I want to think about something else while I am having treatment done.

- When they talk to me about my child's treatment, do they address my child as well? My children tend to take the recommendations more seriously when the dentist and team attempt to make them responsible for their teeth.

- Does the dental team let me know where I am supposed to be during my child's visit? Sometimes I wonder if I should come to the back or if I am allowed. And if I don't come to the back, be sure to tell me and/or show me what was done and what is next. It would be great if they could show me pictures in a consultation room (before and after).

- Are the appointment cards professional and easy to read?

- Do they offer e-mail, text, and phone reminders for appointments?

- Do they offer early, late, or Saturday appointments to fit my work schedule?

- Do they have things that appeal to me, as well as children of various ages? Coffee, water, magazines for adults, age appropriate books and toys for children, and in today's world, wireless Internet for all of us?

- Do they show me what is going on with my mouth, as well as my children's mouths, with x-rays and, especially, photographs?

- Do they explain our dental needs and treatment in a way that is easy to understand?

- Are they nice and friendly to me and my children? Do they seem happy to be at work and happy to see us?

- Is the office clean? (From the reception area to the treatment room, and everywhere in between, moms are looking for neatness and cleanliness. This includes restrooms!)

- Does the team pay attention to me, even when the dentist isn't around?

We've addressed the visual as well as a few of the experiential components of the patient's first impression upon entering the practice. Next we must address the topic of the "new patient experience." Remember, marketing is the message you are sending and the patient is influenced at the highest level on the first visit. If you are taking the time to read this book, I must assume that you want your practice to stand out from the competition and the way that "dental offices usually do things."

Let's outline the ideal new patient experience. Our new patient, Mrs. Jones, arrives at the office twenty to thirty minutes prior to her chair time. While we sent her the link to complete the new patient paperwork, and mailed her a copy, we anticipate that all may not be complete or she may have questions prior to all of her information being finalized.

Mrs. Jones is cheerfully greeted and the scheduling coordinator, Suzanne, introduces herself. She asks Mrs. Jones for her paperwork as it doesn't appear to be submitted online. Mrs. Jones hands Suzanne the paperwork. Suzanne asks Mrs. Jones if she brought her dental benefit card. Mrs. Jones hands Suzanne the card, and Suzanne directs Mrs. Jones to the coffee pot and bottled water. Suzanne lets Mrs. Jones know that they have allowed time at the first visit to establish her electronic chart, and they will be entering her information and verifying her dental benefit coverage.

Within ten minutes, Judy, the financial coordinator, comes to the reception area and introduces herself to Mrs. Jones. She then gives Mrs. Jones a brief tour of the office, introducing her to team members and dentists they encounter along the way, and then shows her to the consultation room, where she reviews Mrs. Jones's information and health history to be sure that all of the information has been entered correctly. Judy assures Mrs. Jones that she will love the practice and that the dentists there are the best in town. She asks Mrs. Jones if she has any questions and answers those for her. Judy then reviews the office confirmation protocol and appointment policy with Mrs. Jones. She offers Mrs. Jones a choice of e-mail, text, and/or telephone confirmation and explains to her the importance of being on time and keeping scheduled appointments. She lets Mrs. Jones know that a twenty-four hour notice is required for cancellations, and Mrs. Jones says she completely understands.

Judy radios Tina, the hygiene assistant, and the dentist that Mrs. Jones is scheduled to see and lets them know that Mrs. Jones is ready. Tina meets Mrs. Jones and Judy in the consultation room and escorts Mrs. Jones to the hygiene operatory. Tina asks Mrs. Jones about her dental health and goals, and Dr. Smith enters the operatory.

He is smiling and is sure to be mask and glove free. He shakes Mrs. Jones' hand and introduces himself. Without taking a seat, he asks Mrs. Jones if she brought x-rays with her or had them sent. She did not. Dr. Smith puts on gloves and takes a quick look into Mrs. Jones's mouth (again, Dr. Smith is standing, not sitting). Dr. Smith tells Mrs. Jones he would like a full mouth set of x-rays so they can establish the condition of not only her teeth but also her gums and bone. Dr. Smith lets Mrs. Jones know he will be back in later to conduct her exam.

Tina takes the x-rays ordered by Dr. Smith and continues in conversation with Mrs. Jones while importing the images into her chart. Next, Tina lets Mrs. Jones know she is going to do a tour of her mouth and gather some images for Dr. Smith to review with her. Tina positions the screen so that Mrs. Jones can see the pictures that are being captured with the camera, and Tina points out areas that may be of concern. Mrs. Jones asks a few questions and Tina makes notes so that Dr. Smith can be sure to answer those questions for her. Tina radios Julie the hygienist and lets her know that Mrs. Jones is ready for her. Julie comes into the room and introduces herself. Tina stays in the room and charts with Julie while she performs periodontal probing. Tina then lets Mrs. Jones know it was nice to meet her and leaves the room. Julie radios Dr. Smith and lets him know that Mrs. Jones is ready. While Julie waits for Dr. Smith, she looks at the x-rays as well as Mrs. Jones's mouth and charts existing restorations as well as makes notes of areas of concern.

Dr. Smith returns to the treatment room and sits down with Mrs. Jones. Before putting on gloves or a mask and before diving into the clinical record, he asks Mrs. Jones, "What's most important to you regarding your dental health?" Mrs. Jones states that she would like to keep her teeth as long as she can. Dr. Smith says, "That sounds like an excellent goal. Let's see what we can do to work with you to achieve it." Dr. Smith asks Julie to pull up the intra-oral images. He reviews those as well as the x-rays with Mrs. Jones and then gloves up to do the evaluation in her mouth. He makes remarks to Julie and Julie mentions the areas of concern that Mrs. Jones had mentioned. Dr. Smith asks Julie to take a few more intra-oral photographs and then raises up the back of the chair so that he and Mrs. Jones are on the same level. He shows Mrs. Jones the x-rays again, several of the images, and also the full-color periodontal chart in their practice management system.

Dr. Smith explains the findings and recommends treatment. Mrs. Jones says she is ready to get started as soon as possible. Dr. Smith recommends a traditional prophy for Mrs. Jones and says he looks forward to seeing her in the next few weeks to start her treatment. Julie scales and polishes and schedules Mrs. Jones for her next hygiene Recare appointment. When the cleaning is complete, Julie escorts Mrs. Jones back to the consultation room and tells her Judy will be with her in a moment.

Judy enters the room and asks Mrs. Jones, "How did it go?" Mrs. Jones talks about how nice everyone is and what a thorough exam Dr. Smith did. Judy says, "Yes, Dr. Smith is wonderful. He is one of the best dentists around." Now Judy pulls up the images with the areas that need treatment and shows Mrs. Jones what Dr. Smith would like to do first. She reviews the fees for the treatment plan and asks Mrs. Jones if she has any questions. Next Judy asks Mrs. Jones, "Would you prefer to pay in full for the upcoming treatment and receive a pre-payment discount or would you like to hear about payment options?" Mrs. Jones says she would like to hear about payment options. Judy finds the best option for Mrs. Jones, and she schedules to begin her work the following Thursday. Judy gives Mrs. Jones her card and asks her to call if she has any questions. Judy then tells Mrs. Jones, "We appreciate having patients like you in our office. It's always a pleasure to see you. And we would love to have more patients just like you. If you have friends or family members looking for a dentist, we would love to take care of them." Mrs. Jones thanks her and leaves the office feeling very impressed.

That evening when Mrs. Jones gets home, her cell phone rings. It's Dr. Smith. He has called her on his way home to let her know how nice it was to meet her. Mrs. Jones feels great about her decision to see Dr. Smith and thinks this will be her dental office for many years to come.

CHAPTER 8

Turn Your Team into a Marketing Machine

W hile external advertising is becoming more important and necessary in today's dental marketplace, we must first focus on marketing to our patient base. There are three primary times when an existing patient will refer to your practice:

1. **After their new patient appointment.** The experience in your office is new and exciting, and if they like you, they are primed to tell others.

2. **When they have completed cosmetic work.** Whether they have whitened their teeth, had bonding, or a complete smile makeover, they want to show off their new smile.

3. **When you have relieved their pain or done something extraordinary.** If you've

worked them in, taken care of their pain, or "removed the thorn from their paw," they will be grateful and want to tell others.

One of the biggest mistakes dental teams make is "not asking for referrals." We hear lots of reasons why...

- We forget to do it.

- It is uncomfortable.

- It doesn't work.

- We sound self-promoting.

As Zig Ziglar would say, "All of those reasons are stinkin' thinkin.'" Your patients and your team are the best promoters and marketers of your practice. We must make it easy for your team and your patients to promote your practice. One of the easiest ways is by using Share A Smile referral cards. This is a small card similar to a business card with your contact information on the front. The back of the card will have text similar to this:

We love our patients and welcome their friends and family. Refer a friend and they will receive a Complimentary New Patient Exam and X-rays.

One time offer valid for new patients only

Many offices have taken the Share A Smile card concept to the next level. We already mentioned that your team members are some of the best marketers for your practice. In addition, we live in a competitive and high tech time; it is no longer cost prohibitive for a dental practice to provide printed business cards for each team member. What better way to promote the practice than to have dental business cards for each team member that also share the role of Share A Smile cards?

Depending on your state practice act, you may be able to state on the card that the referring patient will receive a referral gift or be entered into a drawing. In most states, the promise of a referral reward violates the state practice act. Be sure to check the rules in your state. (Check your state's dental practice act at least once per year for updated advertising guidelines. Be sure to follow those guidelines and adapt our suggestions to fit them.)

I want to emphasize that it is perfectly acceptable to ask for referrals and to make an offer to the new patient. The tricky issue is whether you can promise an incentive to the existing patient for referring their friends and family. In states where the referral incentive for the referring patient is prohibited, you can always send a handwritten, heartfelt thank-you note. And in many cases, you may send an occasional referral reward; you just cannot state or imply that rewards will be given for each referral.

You and your team should be proud of your office, your dentistry, and your fees. There should be no shame at all in thanking a patient for continuing to choose your office (remember, they choose you again each time they return to your office) and letting them know that if they have friends or family members looking for a dentist, you would love to have them join your dental family.

Here's the other beautiful part of patient referrals. People who are great patients—pay their bills, keep their appointments, etc.—tend to refer people who are similar to them. So, this makes this script even better. The following can be said by doctor or team: "Mrs. Jones, we appreciate having patients like you in our office. It's always a pleasure to see you. And we would love to have more patients just like you. If you have friends or family members looking for a dentist, we would love to take care of them."

Then hand the patient two Share A Smile cards. Yes, it is important to hand the cards to the patient because you want them to treat the cards as valuable. Having a stack of them at the front counter or placing them in each take-home dental hygiene goodie bag is not the same. Treat the Share A Smile cards as an item of value and make that clear when you give it to them.

Having the referral conversation and handing out Share A Smile cards is an area where we must be intentional and deliberate. One of the best ways to do this is to choose patients to give Share A Smile cards to during the morning huddle. When we decide in advance who we want to talk with and give these cards to, then we have a greater chance of being successful.

I am going to go into much greater detail here than would be expected for this topic. Asking for referrals is something that most offices know they should do (optional), but few offices realize they must make this a *mandatory* part of the business day. A few patient referrals will happen naturally if we are doing a great job of dentistry and customer service. Yet, smarter dental business owners realize they must do all they can to accelerate this. A new patient referred by an existing patient has a much lower acquisition cost than one acquired by paid advertising. In addition, the referred patients usually stay with the practice and are much more likely to accept treatment and—you guessed it—refer their friends and family.

Here's how to make asking for referrals consistently happen in your practice. Start with these methods and, once you are consistent, you may find alternatives that work better for your practice.

1. Bring a printed schedule, a highlighter, a stack of Share A Smile cards and paper clips to the morning huddle.

2. As you review the schedule, highlight the new patients and choose at least four (or as many as you like) existing patients with whom you plan to have the referral conversation (above).

3. Next, paperclip two Share A Smile cards to the routing slip of each patient with whom you intend to have the referral conversation. This way, the patient will only be given one set of referral cards per visit.

4. After the cards are given, make a note in the dental software system so you will know that you gave the patient Share A Smile cards.

5. Repeat this process each day. This is one of the most important marketing efforts you will have in your office.

What other areas of internal marketing assist in helping your patients to choose you time and time again? Electronic patient communication systems are excellent. These systems interface with your practice management software to communicate with patients via text, e-mail, and/or voice. Not only do these systems send appointment reminders, but they can also be used as a marketing tool to inform patients of additional services you provide, as well as reactivate patients who haven't been in for check-ups or treatment.

Bridge Marketing—The Most Overlooked Marketing Strategies

It seems when we begin to think about external marketing, as well as advertising, we jump straight to thoughts of websites, Facebook, billboards, print ads, direct mail, etc. While these are important to the growth of a practice, there are two bridge marketing strategies that I highly recommend you do before you invest more dollars in the external advertising ventures just mentioned. You may be wondering, what is bridge marketing? It is the area of marketing that is not completely internal or external. It crosses over the gap and fills a unique place in your marketing plan.

It may cross your mind as you read this section that these strategies are old-school, but these particular tried and true methods are the best. Advertising executives spend millions of dollars trying to gain the attention of their prospective customers. They use many different mediums such as television and radio ads, celebrity spokespersons, billboards, social media, Internet ads, and more.

The first step is to thank your referring patients for sending you their friends and family. While it may not be within the realm of your state's practice act to have a referral rewards program, you must remember to thank your referral sources.

Here's why. It's called the law of reciprocation, best outlined in the book *Influence* by Dr. Robert Cialdini. When you do something nice for someone, they feel naturally compelled to do something nice for you. Thus, you would love to create a happy cycle of patients referring to you, you acknowledging them, and this motivating them to refer to you more often.

So here you go, this is my ace-in-the-hole bridge-marketing strategy. Send your patients who refer to you a coffee cup, with your brand and contact information on it, filled with a small arrangement of flowers. Here is the secret component:

Send the arrangement to the referring patient's place of work.

Why is this so powerful? In today's workplace, many things cannot be delivered to the office or place of work. What's the exception in most cases? Flowers.

Here's why sending it to the place of work is such a great idea.

1. Your patient refers their friend, family member, or coworker. They receive the arrangement from your office.

2. Your patient's coworkers ooh and aah that your patient received flowers from their dentist.

CHAPTER 8 | 91

3. This starts a conversation and this is my favorite part of this strategy. coworker to patient, "Wow, your dentist sends you flowers?" Your patient says, "Yes they did. They are letting me know they appreciate me for being a patient and sending referrals." Coworker says, "That's neat. Um, I don't really have a dentist. Is your dentist still seeing new patients? Do you think they would see me?"

4. And in most cases the cycle continues. The coworker becomes a patient and begins to refer their "social network" of friends, family, etc.

The second most powerful bridge marketing strategy is what I refer to as community marketing. Basically, it is community visibility by you (the dentists) and your team. While social media can do some of this for you, I am speaking of face-to-face connections with you, your team, and the community.

I recommend being intentional in this strategy, as well by selecting businesses in the community to "target" with your marketing. This method works in both small-town America as well as the big city. Why? Because, with few exceptions, people love receiving free gifts.

Here's how it works:

1. Create a list of businesses in your community that you wish to market to. I suggest at least one per

week or five per month. Make it easy on yourself
and start with businesses where you already have
patients. Small businesses as well as schools are
usually the most receptive.

2. Place times on the calendar to make visits to these
   area businesses.

3. Decide who in the practice will make visits.

4. Choose what you will deliver. Many practices make
   their own gift baskets and fill them up with goodies
   (food is usually a favorite). This can be snacks,
   breakfast items, toothbrushes. Be creative. And be
   sure to include your Share A Smile cards.

5. Have your designated team member(s), dressed in
   professional office attire (remember they represent
   you and your brand), stop by the local businesses
   with gift basket/goodies in hand.

6. Remind your team that they are out and about in
   the community to create brand awareness and make
   friends.

7. Use social media when it's agreeable by the
   receiving business. Show your team out and
   connecting with community businesses.

8. Be sure to keep a log of the businesses you've visited
   and track monthly stats on where your new patients

are coming from. Your visibility in the community may not pay off immediately, but over time your practice will be known and recognized as a friendly group of caring professionals.

Does the above strategy sound familiar? It's because the dental specialists who are marketing savvy have been marketing to their referral base using these methods for years.

External Marketing and Promotion

This is the area where most practices focus the majority of their marketing attention. Sadly, none of these strategies work well without the internal components in the prior marketing sections in place.

Twenty years ago few dentists advertised their practices. As a matter of fact, when they did, they were frowned upon. Dental advertising has gotten very competitive. Remember the focus of your external advertising needs to be letting the community know you are there and making them aware of any offers you have.

How do most patients find your or any other place of business? Usually they pull out their smartphones and do a search or they look online at their computer. Rarely do your patients even keep their printed phone books and soon they will be a thing of the past.

How do you get started? Remember the patient is buying the brand, and ultimately the dentists. While stock photography is great, having pictures of the dentists, team, and actual patients is a huge benefit. Why? Because anyone can pull photographs of beautiful people and put them on a website, billboard, or direct mail piece. What the patient is looking for is an office with dental professionals they can trust.

You may be thinking, you don't want to have your picture taken or be displayed in your promotions, but this is another time when you have to think like a patient. Remember who makes most of the choices in selecting a healthcare provider—it's women. And women want to know who they are seeing. Do you look like someone they can trust?

Invest in having nice professional photos taken and be sure you prepare ahead of time. Hair, makeup, and clothing selection are very important. You want to look your best. Think about all of the planning that goes into a special event like a wedding. While a photo shoot doesn't have this magnitude, if you have a sizeable marketing budget, these images will be displayed on print and digital media you will spend thousands of dollars on each year. Make it count.

What's most important when it comes to advertising? Meaning if you have a limited budget, where do you start?

95

That's easy: your practice website. It should be easy to navigate. Again, be sure the dentists are easily visible. Also, display before-and-after shots of your own work. Patients want to know that they can trust you to do good work. Also, be sure it has a mobile component or add one. If someone types in your web address on their smartphone, they should not have to squint and try to navigate your entire full-size site on their tiny screen. Be sure your mobile site gives your phone number, map, photos of the doctors, and information patients look for first.

What would be my next recommendation? Direct mail. It's making a comeback. Why? So many companies stopped doing it because of the expense and focused solely on an online strategy. The key with direct mail is the quality of the marketing piece, the offer (yes you need to make an offer), and consistency. Direct mail must be done monthly or quarterly to have an impact.

And if there continues to be room in the marketing budget, the next choices will be online ads and services like Groupon.

But remember: there is no magic pill. There is no slam dunk, no this-is-the-only-marketing-strategy-you-will-ever–need strategy. It's a competitive marketplace. You need to be personally visible in the community, online, and in print.

Section IV

ENGAGEMENT TOOLS

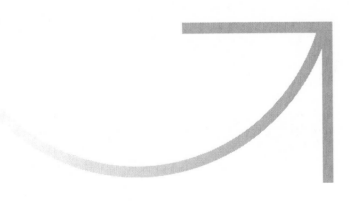

CHAPTER 9

Increasing Your Active Patient Base Through Engagement

Nothing tells your patient quicker that they are not important than your lack of focus on them. Many dentists think that patients leave their practice for two primary reasons: insurance participation and fees. In most cases, the patient either doesn't feel appreciated or doesn't feel the value they receive for services equals the money they are paying. What makes patients feel unappreciated? The reasons include not being greeted promptly and cheerfully, not being seen on time, or watching a team that is more interested in each other than they are in the patients. It all comes down to this—*value*. Patients need to feel valued and they need to see the value in what they are having done. The dental teams who accomplish this have far greater success with patient retention than their competitors.

Let's start with focusing on the patient, making them feel valued while they are in the chair, as well as when they aren't physically present in the office. I like to use the SMILE brand of customer service while the patient is in the office, and we'll call it Smileosophy.

Say the Patient's Name

Make the Patient Feel Important

I Am in Charge of My Attitude

Listen to Your Patients

Exceed Your Patient's Expectations Through Involvement

Say the patient's name as soon as you see him/her. Be sure to use it several times while the patient is in the office. Why? A person's name is the sweetest sound they will ever hear. Wonder how you can significantly impact your long-term or new patients? Make the extra effort to call them by name. Take their photos and have them visible in their records so you can take a look before they come in to make it easier to use their names. Also, tell your patients you appreciate them and thank them for choosing your office. It isn't difficult, but few offices do it consistently. Be intentional and make it happen.

Make the patient feel important by focusing on them. One of the best companies to illustrate how to set the tone for patient focus is Disney. I had the opportunity a few years ago to do one of the behind-the-scenes tours at the Magic Kingdom in Orlando, and for a few hours, I was an honorary cast member. We were instructed that while we were on stage—in sight or earshot of a guest— we were to create an environment that made them feel comfortable and experience the magic. This meant our appearance, our conversations, and our behavior was to support the guest's experience in the park. In the dental office, this means that while the patient is in the practice, we focus on them as much as possible. It also means we do things like put our cell phones out of sight and sound, speak positively of team members and patients, and involve the patient in communication whenever possible.

There are many ways to make the patient feel important outside of the practice as well. If they haven't been in for some time, don't just call them to sell them another appointment. Call them to reconnect and let them know you miss them. Yes, call them. Patient reminder systems are awesome, but sending a text, e-mail, or voice mail reminder is not the same as a connection. Don't overlook the human component. Also, look for opportunities to acknowledge patients. For example, send a card to congratulate them on an engagement, graduation, or other special event.

I am in charge of my attitude. This is probably the component with the most power as it drives the decisions and behaviors of the dentists and everyone on the team. Every day we choose whether we will be happy and grateful or bitter and resentful about our profession, reimbursement, cranky coworker, or patient. Of course, we will all have challenges in life, and there may be days or weeks in our season of life that it's difficult to focus on the positive. Yet, what is the ongoing theme of our life? If you want a better response from your patients or team, start with your attitude. Choose to be at work and be present with your team and your patients—and choose to be happy to be there. It isn't easy, but it is totally worth it. It costs you no more to be happy than it does to be cranky and resentful. Have team members with bad attitudes? Ask yourself why. If their bad attitude is an ongoing occurrence, talk with your team member about it. If it doesn't improve, you cannot afford to keep them.

Listen to your patients. Most people aren't great listeners. Ask your patients what is most important to them and what their goals are, and then listen. Ask them how they have been and what is going on in their life that they are excited about, and then listen. One of the best things you can do when a patient is talking is to make eye contact with them. Sure, we want to work to be efficient, but it only takes a few moments of making eye contact and engaging in conversation to go a long way. This is not only true for the dentist, but also for every team member. Make an effort to listen and be interested in your patients.

Exceed your patient's expectations through involvement. The best way to involve patients in their treatment choices and the value they receive is to show them what you see. Don't simply just show them x-rays. As a former dental office manager, I can promise you most patients don't understand a lot of what an x-ray shows. Show them photos. Don't make the mistake of thinking that these photos need to be of such quality they impress your peers. Whether you use a digital camera or intraoral camera, show the patients their current condition. In today's marketplace, there is no reason not to show the patients their condition at each visit, and also show them their finished product with intraoral photos. Offer to print out copies for them. Patients don't really have the ability to judge quality dentistry; they can only judge customer service. Show them the great work you have done and give them more perceived value for their time and money spent in your practice.

In addition to providing great service in the office, don't overlook the power of staying connected between visits. Dentistry is a relationship business unless we decide that we only want to compete on price, and then it becomes a commodity. Because you are reading this book, I will take it that you want to deepen your patient relationships.

Not to say that social media, e-mail newsletters, and text messages aren't effective in communicating with patients, because they are. However, they don't really enhance the relationship. Only face-to-face and voice-to-voice communication really has that impact. All of the other efforts simply support the person-to-person communication.

Let's highlight some of the best ways to stay engaged with your patients when they aren't physically in the office.

Post-Procedure Calls: While we all know these should be done, I want to share a story that truly hit home with me after a healthcare visit of my own. Because of my travel schedule, I don't always have availability to visit the doctor when I get the occasional sinus infection. So, on a Sunday afternoon, I made my way to my local pharmacy to their "walk-in clinic." I saw a nurse practitioner that completed a thorough exam and sent my prescriptions over to the pharmacy a few feet away. My total bill was $68. I picked up my medicine and proceeded to take it as directed over the next few days. My antibiotic prescription was for five days. On day four, someone from the friendly doc-in-the-box called me. She wanted to know how I was feeling since my prescription was due to run out the next day. I told her I was much better and thanked her for her call. She said, "No problem. If your symptoms return, please come back to see us or see your regular physician."

I hung up the phone and was a little dumbfounded because I received better service and attention from the quick clinic at the pharmacy than I got from my regular physician's office. Hard to believe, isn't it? But it awakened me to the opportunity available to all dental practices and that is to make their patients feel so cared for that they wouldn't dream of leaving.

Evening or next day follow-up calls: Make same-day or next-day calls to patients who had treatment done, as well as to new patients. The post-op calls can be done for any procedure that required an injection or you may choose to contact only those who had certain procedures such as periodontal treatment, root canals, crowns, oral surgery, orthodontic banding, etc. For general, specialty, and other practices that do conscious or IV sedation, contact all sedated patients. Who should make these calls? It is ideal for the dentist to make at least a portion of them. Next best is the clinical team member who assisted with the procedure.

Post seat calls: Many significant procedures might not require a post-op visit. This could include, but is not limited to, crown or bridge seats. While it's impressive to call the same day or next day to be sure they are doing well after the procedure, what will really knock their socks off is a call two to three weeks after the fixed prosthetic is seated.

Concern calls: Most offices have a system in place for calling patients about outstanding treatment plans or unscheduled hygiene Recare appointments by running outstanding treatment reports or Recare reports. Few offices make it a habit to check on patients who haven't been in to simply connect with them. If a patient has items on a treatment plan that are more than nine months old or they are at three months past due for their hygiene recall we want to be sure we let them know we are concerned about them and check on them to see how they are doing. The purpose of this is to have them feel they are important, as well as to let them know you appreciate them and that you miss them. You can also use this opportunity to ask them how they are and if they have any updates to their health history or contact information. Then ask them if there is anything you can do for them. This opens up the door to discuss their current condition and having them schedule their needed treatment or hygiene Recare.

In addition, some of the best opportunities for engagement are when you hear that patients aren't returning to your practice. This is a time when the business owner should take action. If a patient leaves your practice for any reason, the best person to contact them is you. More than likely you spend thousands of dollars a year to attract new patients and not a lot to keep them.

If a patient leaves you for insurance reasons, call them even if you have no intention of getting on their plan. You want to let them know they are important to you, and if they ever decide to come back, you would love to have them. Afraid they will ask you why you don't take their plan? Be honest with them. If you are considering it, let them know. If you aren't considering taking that plan in the near future, let them know that as well, and let them know why. Don't make it about money or quality. Make it about choice. When you commit to becoming a plan provider, you give up the ability of choice for both you and the patient, in many cases, based upon the plan's provisions. It isn't simply a potential reduction in reimbursement. It's that the plan dictates what is covered and treatment options.

If a patient leaves you for any reason other than insurance or moving, call them as well. They likely have great information for you. Maybe there was a situation that occurred once or multiple times in your practice that you aren't aware of. This is a great opportunity for you to listen. If they had a bad experience, apologize. You can apologize even if you weren't aware of the situation or don't have all the facts. Tell them you are sorry that they had a bad experience, and if appropriate, offer to make it right.

Remember, the ultimate goal of patient engagement is to grow your active patient base. This number should be measured a minimum of once per quarter; but for the sake of consistency, most of my clients measure it monthly. Contact your PMS (Practice Management System) company to find out how to run a report showing how many of your active patients have had their last visit in the past twenty-four months. Don't simply go by the number of active patients the PMS tells you that you have. This simply shows how many patients in the database that are flagged as active. It doesn't give a time frame.

CHAPTER 10

Increase Hygiene Membership

This chapter will be of greatest interest to general, pediatric, and periodontal practices. In prior chapters, we have discussed growing the patient base. Now we are going to look at how to increase the number of patients who are active in the hygiene department.

I like to think of the hygiene department as the Hotel California. We want patients to "check in," or join the Recare program, and we never want them to leave. I like to refer to it as "Recare" versus "Recall." We are bringing in the patient to care for them again. Outside of the dental office, a "Recall" is something bad that happens to a vehicle or appliance.

How often should patients be seen for a dental "cleaning" (prophylaxis or periodontal maintenance)? Mouthhealthy. org, the patient-centered website by the American Dental Association, says it's one to three times per year. We know it could be up to four times for some patients, and yet other patients wear dentures and may not be seen at all on the hygiene side. So, let's go with the most common Recare sequence, which is two times per year.

Let's look at how to measure Hygiene Recare Effectiveness, or Hygiene Membership. The most accurate rule of thumb is to review the number of Recare exams compared to active patients and compute a ratio.

First, let's look at how many periodic exams we conduct over a year's time. For this example, let's say that 1,320 periodic exams were performed over the last twelve months. (This figure can be found on a detailed report of production by procedures in your PMS.)

Next, let's find the number of patients that are active in the practice. Again, don't go by the figure that the PMS shows as active because it contains everyone who isn't flagged inactive. Run a report showing how many patients had their last visit within twenty-four months. In this example, we will use the figure of 2,000 active patients; and if they potentially need two Recare visits per year, that's a total of 4,000 potential Recare visits needed.

Divide the current number of Recare visits performed – 1,320

By the potential Recare visits needed (based on Active Patients x 2) – 4,000

Which is a 33 percent Recare Effectiveness rate in Hygiene Membership

Unfortunately, 33 percent is the average for practices who don't intentionally work on this area of the practice. But the great news is you can achieve much higher participation in Hygiene Membership and hygiene production by implementing the following systems.

Be sure everyone in the practice is on the same page regarding recommended Recare sequence. To fully engage the patient in the importance of why they need to come in to the practice for recommended Recare visits, the entire team must support the doctor in discussing with the patient, ideally at their first visit, how often they recommend for that individual patient to come in and why. Yes, the hygienist and rest of the team should reinforce it, but it matters the most when it comes from the dentist. The hygienist or assistant should prompt the dentist by asking, "How often would you like to see Mrs. Jones for a cleaning?" This gives the dentist the opportunity to prescribe the Recare sequence in front of the patient and explain why that sequence fits their needs. It also makes the patient feel there is a reason for how often they should come in, instead of "being due for a cleaning because insurance will pay for it."

Adopt the mindset that each patient should leave with their next hygiene appointment scheduled. In other words, you want every patient in hygiene to commit to their next Recare visit before they leave today's visit. There is one exception. Do not pre-appoint "repeat offenders." What is a repeat offender? A patient or family of patients who have cancelled short notice or broken several appointments in the past. Those patients should be sent a reminder card to schedule when their Recare visit is due. This prevents 80 percent of the last minute openings in the hygiene schedule.

Please ignore the articles you have read about avoiding pre-appointing in hygiene. I have been in dozens of practices first-hand who have followed this poor advice. I believe the reasoning behind it is to reduce last minute cancellations. I am sure it does reduce them, but it misses the larger picture of having more patients active in hygiene, more hygiene production, more diagnosis for operative, and more operative production. The offices I have worked with that stopped pre-appointing hygiene had decreases in hygiene production of 33 to 50 percent in less than twelve months.

Pre-appointing works, but you must carefully follow the recommended sequence.

The best location in the office to make the next hygiene appointment is in the hygiene room, while the patient is still seated. Once the Recare sequence has been established and while making this a new habit, go ahead and schedule the patient for their next hygiene visit at the beginning of the appointment. Rarely will it need to be moved based upon the doctor's recommendation unless the patient has had a significant change in their health or oral hygiene. The primary reason to have the patient schedule with their hygienist or hygiene assistant is that once the patient is up and out of the chair, they are ready to go. We want to make this a priority and be sure it is done before the patient arrives at the counter to checkout.

Add to your preparation for the next day's morning huddle, a review of patients for the day:

- Who have never been seen in hygiene for Recare.

- Who are past their recommended time sequence for Recare.

- Who have immediate family members (spouse, children, etc.) who aren't currently scheduled for Recare.

Most clients find it is most effective to either make a note of this on the schedule or on the routing slips for review in the morning huddle. Be intentional about discussing the need for their cleaning and exam, and you will be surprised that several appointments per day will be made because of the focus on this information. In addition, you are likely to be able to go ahead and see a few of those patients that day if your schedule allows.

One of the best tools you can add to your practice is an automated appointment reminder system. These software add-ons can alert you to who needs to be called that day or month for their Recare visits. Then you can send text messages or e-mail messages to invite the patients to schedule. These automated patient engagement systems are wonderful for patients who have been in recently (less than twelve months). Beyond that time frame, it is best to make direct contact with the patient, letting them know they are missed.

Who are the best people on the team to contact patients who haven't responded to initial contacts regarding scheduling their Recare visit? Initially, either an administrator or clinical team member can make the calls. If after the first efforts, there is no response from the patient, have their preferred hygienist give them a call, letting them know they are missed. The patient will already know they are past due for their recommended

Recare, so let them know we are concerned about them and miss them.

Now, for the patients who pre-appointed, what is the best way to remind them of their appointments while also keeping last minute changes to a minimum? Many offices that have been using an automated appointment reminder system for some time, no longer send postcards. At this time, most practices still mail a reminder or confirmation card. So here is an outline of how the confirmations should work:

1. Two weeks prior to the appointment, mail the postcard or send the reminder by e-mail or text.

2. One week prior to the appointment, make a week-ahead call or electronic reminder. It simply says, "Jim, we are reaching out to be sure that your hygiene appointment scheduled for next week on Tuesday at 10 a.m. still works for you. Is there anything that might prevent you from keeping this appointment?" Basically, you want to know a week out if they need to make a schedule change.

3. Now we will do a day-before call or electronic reminder, letting Jim know we are looking forward to seeing him tomorrow at 10 a.m.

The secret to making pre-appointed Recare work is the week-ahead contact. Think about it: how much sense does it make to only mail a card for an appointment made six months ago and then call the patient a day or two before? Of course, some of them may have missed the postcard and now you have an appointment to fill on short notice. The week-ahead direct contact gives you an ample window to easily reschedule the patient's appointment, if needed.

In order to be sure that your team is compliant with pre-appointing, use your PMS system to forecast how many appointments are scheduled or how much production is scheduled in four, five, and six months. In other words, in the month of January, look at the hygiene appointments scheduled for April, May, and June. This number should be at least 90 percent of the average number of Recare exams per month.

Combine Recare pre-appointments with the appropriate confirmation sequence, maintain your daily focus on being sure that each patient in the practice has their next Recare visit scheduled, and utilize your PMS to connect with your patients who are past due for their recommended hygiene sequence, and you will watch your Hygiene Membership numbers grow.

CHAPTER 11

Increasing Case Acceptance

"Every sale has five basic obstacles: no need, no money, no hurry, no desire, and no trust."

— Zig Ziglar

Having a profitable practice is much easier to achieve when more patients say "yes" to dentistry. This is especially true as dentists continue to receive lower rates of reimbursement from dental plans with stagnant annual maximums. This means, in most cases, that patients have to pay more out of pocket than ever before. So our job as dental professionals is to communicate with our patients in a manner that reveals what they really want for their health, and show them how to get it.

The foundation of case acceptance is identity of the dentist and his/her team. Identity answers the question who am I? For your practice it goes deeper: Who are we? What type of care do we believe our patients want? How will we deliver that care?

To simplify this concept, if you believe patients want the best for their oral health you will interact with them in a way that matches those beliefs. Or if you believe that patients only want what is less expensive, or what insurance will pay for, that is how you will present their conditions and recommended treatment.

Next your identity is represented in what you talk about in your marketing and how the practice is represented or communicated. Your style and how you communicate your clinical skill—meaning appearance, communication skills, and appeal—are more important to the patient initially than your actual clinical skill. Now allow me to be clear, style without the training and skill level to back it up is dangerous and will make for a short-lived reputation. The point I am aiming for is excellence in clinical skills is not enough. Patients assume that all dentists are skilled because the dental schools graduated them and gave them a license.

Another significant component is likeability. This term was newly introduced in the last decade in business, primarily due to the boom in social media. Yet likeability isn't limited to an online or onscreen audience. Patients decide whether or not they like or trust you based on the following:

- Is your appearance professional, neat, and clean?

- Do you make eye contact with them?

- Do you make efforts to get in rapport with them by showing a sincere interest in them, listening to them, and focusing more on them than on your teammates, or perish the thought, your smartphone? (Your smartphones should never be visible to a patient in the practice.)

- Do you work to match their communication style? If the patient is high energy and talks fast, you and your team should work to communicate to them in a way that matches their body language, tone of voice, and speed of speech. Or if a patient is more on the quiet and meek side, you may need to lower your voice and slow your speech down a bit to match theirs. The simplest way to achieve this is to watch your patients and focus on getting in sync with their communication style.

Likeability comes naturally for many people and is something others must work at. The good news is, likeability can be worked upon and improved. It may seem a bit stiff or unnatural but the main component to remember is that you want to develop and improve upon how you come across to others in order to continuously improve how well you, your team, and your message are received.

Therefore how you and your team communicate, both verbally and non-verbally, sends a direct message to your patients about the type of care that is delivered in your practice.

Here are some questions to ask yourself regarding the message your practice is sending:

- What does my Internet presence say about my practice?

- What does my facility say about the quality of care in our office?

- What does my appearance and the appearance of our team say about our professionalism and how we work together?

Many times patients will fall out of a buying mode simply because the brand of the practice, the environment of the facility, or the interaction with the team is a turn-off. To reinforce, identity is to case acceptance what bone level and gum tissue are to teeth. It is a vital aspect and must be in great shape to support what is visible.

Beyond identity, the greatest success in case acceptance hinges on two methods or skills:

1. Our ability to discover what the patient wants, listen to them, and communicate their treatment options in such a way to let them know which route will best help them reach their goals. In other words, we must discover their goals, wants, wishes, values, and sense of urgency regarding their oral health. The bottom-line: we must be great at asking the right questions, listening, and then helping the patients make the best decision.

2. Equally important to our communication ability is the use of intraoral images to show patients the condition of their mouth. The intraoral camera not only engages patients in their oral health and gives them ownership of their condition, it builds trust because they can see what you see. Sadly, many offices have cameras but they are either not functioning or grossly underutilized. In most cases, the camera or intraoral photos should be used with 80 percent of your patients, at every visit. It's time to raise our standards and become consistent with utilizing the camera.

Communication Is Key

We must make the following statement part of our core beliefs when interacting with patients: Every chart or patient record has a name; every name has goals, wants, wishes, values, and a time frame regarding their decisions relating to their oral health. In other words, every patient has a "smile story." We must learn to uncover it. To do so, we begin chair-side with the following conversation:

> "Mrs. Smith, what is most important to you in your oral health?" *Listen*
>
> Next, if she doesn't address it, ask her:
>
> "How long would you like to keep your teeth?" *Listen*
>
> "Are there any other goals you would like for us to be aware of?" *Listen*
>
> "Is there anything else you would like for us to know, or anything you wish were different about your smile?" *Listen*

In most instances where treatment is not accepted it wasn't the lack of explanation regarding the needed procedures that prevented you from making the sale, it was the lack of involvement in including the patient in their goals and values for their treatment.

Now let's take it to the next level and talk about team communication hand-offs. Just like the importance of a smooth connection with the baton in a relay race, we must be sure the thread of communication isn't dropped as the patient has exchanges between departments and also with their dentist.

Where are communication hand-offs needed? Every instance where the patient is being communicated with regarding their needs or proposed treatment, or in front of more than one team member. Communication hand-offs begin when the patient goes from the administrative team to the clinical team. Next, the communication flows from the clinical assistant or hygienist to the doctor. Toward the end of the appointment there should be a hand-off conversation from the doctor back to the clinical assistant or hygienist and then from that team member to the administrative team.

Here is an example of exactly how the communication hand-off works:

1. **"Welcome."** The administrative team makes eye contact and greets the patient by name. "Hello Mrs. Smith. It is great to see you today. Our clinical team will be with you shortly." That administrative team member alerts the appropriate department, either by computer or verbally, that Mrs. Smith has arrived.

2. **"What we are doing today."** The dental assistant or hygienist escorts the patient to the back and seats the patient. While making eye contact, she says to the patient, "Mrs. Smith, your chart shows that we are doing a crown on tooth #2 today and a tooth colored filling on tooth #3. Let me show you a photo of the area we are working on. Do you have any questions before we get started?" The patient may have a question or two and the assistant readily answers, and then she makes the patient comfortable and applies a topical anesthetic. Now, when the doctor enters the operatory the assistant says, "Dr. Jones, I have everything ready for the crown prep on tooth # 2 and the composite on tooth #3 for Mrs. Smith and I have shown the photos to her. She is ready to get started." Then the doctor greets the patient, gives anesthesia, and returns in a few moments to begin the procedure. Or if a hygienist is numbing the patient, the assistant will have this conversation as the doctor enters the room, is getting their gloves on, and is sitting down.

3. **"What we completed today."** Once Mrs. Smith's crown on tooth #2 and filling on tooth #3 are completed and the doctor is finishing his duties in the room, the assistant says, "Dr. Jones, I have notated in Mrs. Smith's chart the crown prep on tooth #2 and the two surface DO composite

on tooth #3. Are there any additional notes you would like for me to make?" She makes the notes and, if appropriate, shows Mrs. Smith a photo of the completed work if the permanent crown was made in-house. If not, plan to show her an after photo at the seat appointment.

4. **"What's next."** The assistant says in front of the patient, "Dr. Jones, Mrs. Smith's treatment plan shows that the next treatment Mrs. Smith needs is to have the crown on tooth #2 seated and to prep the crown on tooth #28, on the lower right." The assistant pulls up a photo of the lower right or takes one with the camera. "Do you recommend that she has both of those procedures done at the same visit?" Dr. Jones replies, "Yes, we can definitely do both of those procedures at the same visit since they are on the same side." The assistant says, "Mrs. Smith, would you like to get the crown prepped on tooth #28 at your next visit?" Mrs. Smith says, "Yes." The assistant responds, "Let's go see Susan and she can schedule that appointment for you and discuss your payment options." Note, if the next treatment weren't being scheduled in conjunction with a seat appointment, the assistant would want to ask the doctor, "Dr. Jones, how soon do you recommend that Mrs. Smith have this crown completed?" This prompts the doctor to let the patient know the

amount of urgency they should consider when making the decision to schedule.

4. **"See you next time."** The assistant escorts Mrs. Smith to the administrative area to talk with Susan, the financial coordinator. The assistant says, "Susan, we completed the crown prep on tooth #2 today and the tooth colored filling on tooth #3 for Mrs. Smith. Dr. Jones would like to do the crown on tooth #28 at the same time we seat the crown on tooth #2, and that will need to be three to four weeks from now. Mrs. Smith, it was great working with you today, and I look forward to seeing you soon. Please let us know if you have any questions between now and your next visit." Mrs. Smith says, "Thank you for everything." The assistant replies, "You're most welcome," and then heads back to the clinical area.

As you can see, team communication hand-offs are so simple; all team members are clearly communicating the patient's needs to each other, and communication is seamlessly carried through from beginning to end. Most importantly, your patient finally has the information they need to make a true commitment to your recommended treatment plan. However, this kind of top-notch communication can't happen without concerted effort, lots of practice, and continual coaching.

The Importance of Intraoral Cameras

Without a doubt, the intraoral camera (or high-end digital camera), is the most underutilized marketing and sales tool you have in your practice. Rarely are these photographs for our benefit. They are to show the patients their current condition, show them the work we have completed—which gives them huge value immediately for their investment—and then show them what is next.

Here are the opportunities to use the camera that your team should attempt to incorporate as habits. If you really want to make this change, make the use of the camera mandatory, even if you must buy more cameras. Ideally you should have an intraoral camera in each operatory. Also realize, x-rays are awesome, yet they are primarily for our use to diagnose. A photograph is something that is easy to understand and requires little explanation when something doesn't look right.

The intraoral camera (or showing the patients previous images) must be used:

- On every new patient.

- On every recall patient with outstanding treatment or with newly diagnosed treatment.

- On every operative patient to show them what tooth or area we are working on today (show them pre-op and when restoration is complete, show them post-op). Use your own judgment—80 percent of post-op images are great to show. If they are coming back in a week or two for a post-op or it's an oral surgery procedure, you may not want to show those images.

- In operative or hygiene, show the patients who have a condition that is worsening how much worse they present today than they did last visit, last year, or whenever the treatment was diagnosed.

Decide in the huddle which patients you will use the camera for and discuss patients who have been delaying treatment. In some cases the reason for the delay may be financial. In other cases, they don't value the work enough to part with the money.

How can you make utilizing the camera a habit in the operatory? Here is a great mantra when adopting a new habit: Do it first—before you switch onto auto-pilot and forget about it. So for new patients, the first thing you should place in their mouth is the camera wand. Start off their visit by engaging them immediately. Let the patient know, "We are going to take a tour of your mouth using our intraoral camera. Along the way, I will show you areas that are good and areas that will be a point of discussion with the doctor. Do you have any questions?"

Another example will be in operative, where a patient, Mr. Crabapple, has returned to have an MO surface composite on tooth #2 and an MOD composite filling on tooth #3. If we already have a photo, we can pull it up on the screen to show Mr. Crabapple what we are working on today, or we can simply show him with the camera. Be sure to capture the image if you don't already have it. At the end of the visit, let him see the "after" photo. This not only gives him confidence in your treatment but it creates value and makes it easier for him to justify the expense when he arrives at the counter to pay.

Financing—How to Have a Money Conversation

It wouldn't be a sales conversation if we didn't talk about the money part. This is often the area that stops dental teams in their tracks. Go back to the beginning of the chapter where we talked about our beliefs. If we believe that patients want the best for their oral health, we won't let their questions or objections about money stop us from effectively working with them to achieve their oral health goals. And we can have the conversations without being pushy or high pressure. We must put on our hat as their dental health coach, and once the patient has decided they want the treatment, the role of the financial coordinator is finding the best payment solution for the patient.

First, your team must be crystal clear about the payment options you offer. It is never recommended that you play the role of the bank. There have never been more options available to assist patients in their cost of care. Be sure to have an option where patients can pay in full prior to treatment or at the first visit of their treatment plan, and receive a 5 percent discount. Next, have options available where the patients can split payments into phases. For example, if treatment is $2,000 and will be spread over six weeks, we could allow that patient to make three equal payments, every two weeks. Every practice should have outside payment plans, which allow the patient to spread their treatment over months, or even years, so they can receive the treatment they want in a way that fits into their budget. The most popular option for that is www.carecredit.com. Lastly, if you want to consider accepting payments from a patient of record with whom you have a great payment history, be sure to use an automatic account debit of either their credit card or bank account. With red flag rules, and the liability you have of having a drawer in the office with little slips that have patient credit card numbers on them, be sure to use a service for this, or ask your bank if this is available. You want the account to be automatically debited each month for the agreed amount, and the card or account information to be encrypted.

Here is a sample script for determining which direction is most appropriate for the patient in paying for their treatment. For this example, we will use a patient who is beginning a new treatment plan.

Mrs. Green, the total for your treatment is $5,000. Would you be more interested in hearing about a discount for paying in full or options for making payments?

> *Note this is an open-ended, not a yes or no, question. We want to avoid asking the patient a question where the answer could be no as it cools off the readiness to commit.*

Now their answer can be one of three things:

- Both.

- I would like to hear about the cash discount.

- I would like to know about the payment plans.

If they answer both or pay up front with a discount, simply say, "We offer our patients a 5 percent discount off of the total amount when they pay in full up front."

If they answer both or that they would like payment plan information, say, "I am happy to tell you about our payment options. Do you have a monthly amount in mind or have you thought about how much time you would want to pay for the treatment?" This gives you a bearing on where to start. If they say they will need twenty-four months, or they can pay $50 per month, then you want to start with a payment plan that fits those particular time frames.

What's most important in these financial conversations is to support the commitment level the patient has for their oral health goals. Also, whenever possible sit next to the patient, rather than across from them, when discussing their payment options.

Last but not least, be sure the patient signs the financial agreement. This happens automatically when you are utilizing an outside payment plan. For any other agreement, including a payment in full with a discount, be sure to have the terms in writing, and have the patient sign it. Then give a copy to the patient and file a copy in your records.

Case acceptance is a team activity and starts before we ever take a look in the patient's mouth. Meet with your team, and discuss your beliefs regarding the type of dentistry patients want, and what you would like to deliver. This will begin to point you in the right direction.

Section V

ORGANIZATIONAL TOOLS

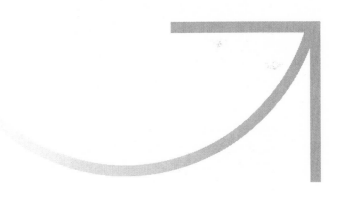

CHAPTER 12

Increasing Efficiency

Time management is a make-or-break system in every dental practice. What's the key? Being sure you and your team manage your schedule and avoid letting your schedule manage you. Smarter Dental Scheduling is a combination of goal setting, planning, delegation, communication, and evaluation. Utilize the following strategies to get your appointment book in shape and schedule smarter in order to reach your goals:

1. Know your daily and hourly goals. The daily production goal must be determined and plugged into the software system. Your ability to reach your production goals is directly related to the knowledge that each and every team member has about the goal for each day. Goals should be broken down by department and chair. For example, in a million dollar practice

working 192 patient contact days per year, the daily goal would be $5,208. In a general practice, at least a third of this goal should be produced by the hygiene department. The daily goal for the hygiene department per day would be $1,720. If the hygiene department were staffed by one hygienist and an assistant or two hygienists, utilizing two rooms, the hygiene goal per day would be $860 per chair. The same formula will work for operative. In the same example of the $5,208 goal for the practice, if the hygiene department goal is $1,720 per day, the operative goal would be $3,488. If the doctor worked out of two rooms with two assistants, the goal would be $1,744 per chair each day.

2. Know your available chair hours and expand when possible. You may wish to refer back to the calculation of chair hour value in the "Knowing Your Numbers" section. Available chair hours are defined as the number of chairs in your practice x the number of hours the practice is open for dentistry. This is particularly critical when there are multiple dentists. A practice can double its capacity, with two or more dentists, by working split schedules. For example, open the office from 7am to 7pm and have each dentist for a six hour schedule. You will have increased overhead in staffing, yet you

keep you fixed costs the same and don't incur additional debt. In addition, you make the practice more available to your patients. Also, as the dental economy becomes more competitive, consider offering weekend hours, if you haven't already added them.

3. Time your clinical procedures. Knowledge is power. Usually an office has an idea of how long a procedure will take and only sometimes is this accurate. By timing your procedures in the practice, and examining doctor, hygiene, and assistant time, you will glean a lot of information about how to not only make the schedule more productive, but also less stressful. As an example, think about professional athletes. They are constantly measuring their progress. Whether it is a race time, distance run, or monitoring their form via video, constant measurement is part of their protocol. The same methods can be used in the dental practice. If you have never timed your procedures before, it isn't too late to start. If you have already timed your procedures, then be sure you are scheduling an annual or semi-annual retiming. With new technologies, materials, and employee turnover it doesn't take much to disturb the balance of your finely tuned schedule.

4. Schedule appointments by "primary" provider time. Each appointment can be broken down into primary and secondary time or doctor/assistant and hygiene/assistant time. The practice only drives revenue at a healthy level when we make sure to schedule around the primary provider's time. In other words, we want the primary providers (doctors and hygienists) scheduled to do the "special things" they went to school for as much as possible. So, if a crown prep takes a total of 80 minutes on the schedule, the doctor's time should only be blocked off during the time in which he or she must be in the room (anesthesia, prepping the crown, impression, etc.). Simply blocking the doctor's column for the 80 minutes is not an effective use of the scheduling system or the doctor's book.

5. Know your state dental practice act. How familiar are you with the state practice act? Recruiting and training a highly qualified team is of utmost importance in your ability to schedule effectively. Hiring decisions should be based on the credentials needed for a hygienist or assistant to function at full capacity. Next, look at the procedures in the practice that have components that could be delegated by the doctor to an assistant or hygienist. Schedule in-house team

training to get all team members up to speed on all skills that the doctor can delegate. Get creative about when you will conduct training. Training does not have to take away from patient care. Not only will this allow the doctor or hygienists to be more productive, but it also makes work more interesting for the clinical team.

6. Create an ideal schedule with a pre-blocked template. If you are truly committed to scheduling for maximum efficiency, then creating a schedule template is the best route. Take your daily goal by department and chair and work with the entire team to lay out the best schedule to allow for quality dentistry and the personal touch while continuing to deliver impeccable care. If you have too many procedures scheduled at the same time, quality and customer service will suffer. Many practices schedule their most difficult procedures, which are often the highest production, in the morning when everyone is fresh and there are fewer interruptions.

7. Establish accountability for the schedule. It is easy to blame the administrative team if the schedule isn't booked productively. While the administrative team has a lot of control over the schedule, their ability to keep a productive schedule can have a lot to do with the support from the clinical team.

There should be one person at the front desk who is primarily accountable for the doctor's schedule and one person at the front desk who is primarily accountable for the hygiene schedule. Every team member plays a part in keeping the schedule productive. As we mentioned earlier, each chair has a goal each day. The team member in charge of that chair should be aware of the schedule for the current and next day.

8. Establish a protocol for handling emergency patients. You've heard the phrase "one man's junk is another man's treasure." Many practices see emergency patients (especially emergency "new" patients) as a headache. Others see them as an opportunity. Develop a protocol for getting emergency patients in the office quickly, evaluating their needs, and rendering treatment or at least getting them out of pain. Even the best orchestrated schedules have changes. Capitalize on the changes in your schedule to accommodate emergency patients and reap the rewards of many new "lifetime" patients.

9. Be flexible about hygiene Recare checks. Many offices have gotten into a rut and wait until the end of the hygiene appointment to page the doctor to come in and check. In busy practices,

this can have the doctor checking three to four hygiene chairs per hour. This many exam requests at the end of every hour is overwhelming and leads to stressed out doctors, hygienists, and patients. Have the hygiene team page the dentist as soon as the patient is seated and charting is done. Encourage the dentists to stop by hygiene whenever possible, in between the "doctor time" of restorative procedures. This allows the doctor to check patients in hygiene when he or she has time and prevents the entire hygiene department from needing their patients checked simultaneously.

10. Develop a high level of communication regarding the schedule. There should be an enormous amount of verbal and written communication each day in the office regarding the schedule. Many offices use devices and technology such as radios, communication lights, or instant messaging systems. Those tools are a great starting point. The type of communication we are talking about is more of a "culture" issue. Just look at great sports teams. Not only are they highly skilled, but they are constantly talking with one another about the next move. There should be the same level of verbal communication in the practice about what the patients need or their next appointment. The pieces of technology can also be very useful in real-time when there is an opening.

A quick radio message or instant message letting everyone know there is an opening the next hour in hygiene or operative yields a much greater chance of the appointment being filled by a patient who is already in the office for another type of procedure.

No other management system in the practice can bring as many rewards or as much stress as the management of the patient schedule. Smarter Dental Scheduling is not only a system but also a continuous process. Understanding the value of time, the importance of how it is utilized, and having a commitment to communicate regarding the opportunities to utilize open time are the keys to reaching your goals and being as profitable as possible. Remember, you are the owner of your schedule, and time is one of your most precious resources. Invest the planning and training to maximize it.

Section VI

BRINGING IT ALL TOGETHER

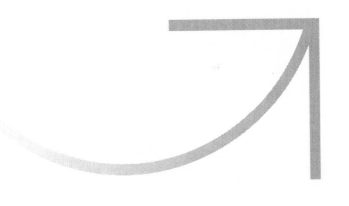

CHAPTER 13

The Importance of Having a Coach

I've had the privilege of coaching dentists and their teams since 1994. Over the last two decades, there have been many changes in the business of dentistry and those changes keep coming faster and faster.

Many of these changes are incredibly positive. Technology has allowed dentists to diagnose and treat patients in ways that are less time consuming for the dentist, as well as more convenient and more comfortable to the patient.

As business owners, there is unlimited access to information via the Internet, dental forums, online articles, and continuing education courses. This is a double-edged sword for the following reasons. First, all of the advice online isn't necessarily good advice or the best advice for your practice. Second, knowing what to do is only part of the equation. Implementing the best systems, communication techniques, and marketing strategies is what counts. Most of the clients I work with who are profitable and also have less amounts of stress aren't striving to "know more." They work every day to become more consistent with what they know works.

There has never been a more critical time in the business of dentistry to have a coach. Maybe you have one or have had one in the past. In my business, I have had periods of time where I have had a coach and where I have not. One of the biggest mistakes I ever made was going without coaching for a period of time. Nothing happened initially to make a negative impact, but slowly I began to become more lax in my accountability to my team and their accountability to me. Systems became more flexible and many disappeared. Why? Well, I was busy and I "knew" what needed to happen. We began to drift slowly off course from our vision and goals. The change was so slow that I really didn't notice it at first. When I did notice, my business needed more than tweaking, it needed resuscitating. So I made the decision that as long as I have my own business, I will have a business coach.

Here are the reasons why having a coach for your dental business is so important (from both the coaching perspective, as well as the business owner perspective):

1. **Perspective.** Because the coach doesn't work "in your business," they see things that you don't see. After you have been in practice for a while, you begin to adjust to how things are and you lose the ability to "see" things that a coach will see. This can be numbers, scheduling inefficiencies, lack of systems, etc. A coach has the perspective to see what's missing between where you are now and your goals and potential.

2. **Higher Ceiling.** A coach sees beyond your current situation into what your practice can be. Because dental business coaches work with a variety of practices, especially if they work with practices with different geographic dynamics, they know what is possible and have seen it work in a variety of environments. A coach can share benchmarks with you and help you go beyond where you thought you were capable of going.

3. **Focuses You on Your Goals, Vision, and Numbers.** A coach's job is to direct their client's focus toward achieving their goals and vision. A coach will assist you in developing your vision and goals that support it. A coach will also insist that you know your numbers. Business decisions are sometimes made on emotion, but if they are sound decisions, they must be justified with facts and numbers. You

cannot compete and thrive in today's dental economy without knowing your numbers better than anyone else in your practice.

4. **Efficiency and Organization.** Based upon your practice and resources, a coach will make recommendations on how you can be more organized and practice more efficiently.

5. **Continual Growth.** Your business is either growing or shrinking. There is no autopilot and no cruise control. We live and work in an economy where you cannot afford to just "keep things the way they are."

6. **Peaks and Valleys.** Every business and business owner has them. There will be mountain top moments and there will be rock bottom times as well. A coach plays an important role on both ends of the spectrum and every step in between. The decisions you make and actions you take when you are experiencing great success determine how long you will stay there, and the same is true for when you are at a low point. For example, business is down, so you pull back on your advertising. Not as many potential patients can find you, which reduces your new business, therefore lowering your production even more.

7. **Trusted Advisor and Confidante.** A coach takes a personal interest in you and believes in you. This is especially important when you are the sole owner or one of a few owners in your group. Sometimes you can feel like you are doing this alone, and it isn't easy. The truth is, it is possible and it doesn't have to be difficult. Sometimes the extra push you need is knowing that someone believes in you and your ability, and they remind you of that.

8. **Challenges You To Continually Improve.** A coach wants more for you. They will listen and challenge you to raise your standards. This may range from improving customer service or case presentation skills to expecting more from your team or assisting you in choosing a higher caliber employee. A great coach will do it in a way that has you know they are doing it because they care, not because they are on a power trip.

In summary, having a coach is like having a personal trainer for your business. Asking for help isn't a sign of weakness, it's a sign of commitment that you are ready for things to get better. You will likely have different coaches for different aspects and phases of your business. How do you know who you should work with? Whether you call and interview me or other business coaches, ask for at least three references. Talk to other business owners who have worked with that coach and ask them if they would hire the coach again and what growth they experienced (in their numbers, leadership, teamwork) from working with them.

Remember, you can do this. Also remember, it's easier and the path is clearer with good coaching for your practice.

CHAPTER 14

Conclusion

While you were in dental school, you undoubtedly had big dreams for your future practice. Are you finding that some of those dreams are as yet unfulfilled? What was it you wanted to accomplish by going into dentistry in the first place? Even if you feel like you've hit a road block, the good news is: you can do it. How do I know? Because others have done it; you simply need to take the time to apply the management tool steps in this book and you can too.

Remember the Five Keys to Growth – be sure you are focusing your strategies in these areas.

1. Increase New Patients

2. Increase Active Patients

3. Increase Hygiene Membership

4. Increase Case Acceptance

5. Increase Efficiency

Management Tools Checklist

☑ Know your numbers. Learn your software system and take time to understand the business reports for the practice.

☑ Set goals that are realistic and based on real information. Have a clear bonus system tied to the goals and involve the team in setting those goals.

☑ Make it easy to become a new patient by booking on the first call and offering free or low-cost exams for first time patients.

☑ Think like a new patient. Does your office environment set them at ease? Is your staff welcoming? Does the office communication style make them feel informed and valued?

☑ Ask for Referrals! Use Share A Smile cards with your valued patients.

☑ Use a combination of internal and external marketing techniques to reach a wide potential patient base. There is no one "best" technique.

☑ Engage your active patients with excellent customer service using the Smileosophy.

☑ Make all patients feel valued and important.

☑ Increase Hygiene Membership by pre-booking appointments and clearly communicating the need for the treatment with patients.

☑ Listen to patients and make sure your brand of communication makes them feel valued. Reinforce that you care about their health and be sure they understand why procedures are being recommended.

☑ Schedule smartly—make sure your time is being used efficiently to create more profitable time on the calendar.

☑ Work with a coach to gain perspective and have outside feedback to help you get to the next level in your growth.

You may be frustrated right now. It may seem no one understands the struggle of managing your practice. But know that many thousands have gone before you and are now experiencing the joy of success. In dental school you learned so much, but you probably never dreamt you had to learn about accounting, marketing, time-management, and even a little psychology. You've taken a great step in starting to learn about the other elements of running your business. But knowledge alone is not enough; you need to apply that knowledge.

Start to take these steps little-by-little. Schedule time on your calendar to work on your business. Reach out to get the help you need—from your own team and from outside sources. You can accomplish more when you reach out for help than trying to go it alone.

If you focus on what needs to be done, month by month, you can succeed. Give it everything you have got. It won't be easy—nothing of importance ever is. Becoming a dentist was not easy, but you focused on that and achieved it. Surround yourself with people who care about your success and manage them properly. Then you will reach your dreams by growing your dental business into something greater than you believed possible.

About the Author

Penny Reed is an expert in the business of dentistry. Her unique combination of management experience, success as a dental practice consultant, and business administration background make her one of the most effective dental business coaches in North America. With more than twenty-three years of experience, Penny has the ability to quickly pinpoint challenges and take any practice to the next level.

In 1992 Penny was recruited by her own dentist to manage his growing dental practice. Penny worked as an office manager in this dental practice and became adept at managing personnel issues, negotiating financial agreements, implementing a scheduling protocol, and developing other must-have skills for successfully running a dental practice. Her excitement about the possibilities for improving struggling or stagnant practices using her proven methods prompted Penny to enter the dental consulting world.

Penny has written hundreds of articles which have been published in such widely read publications as *Dental Economics*, *Dentistry Today*, and *Inside Dentistry*. She was interviewed in the *Learning About Cosmetic Dentistry* series by PBS and has been named a Leader in Dental Consulting by *Dentistry Today* from 2007 to 2016.

Penny works with dentists who want to grow their practices, become more profitable, and have a better quality of life. As a result of her work, her clients are more focused, have more income, more confidence, and have happier teams to support them. On a personal note, Penny loves to make people laugh and has always dreamt of having a talk show. She lives with her husband and two daughters in Collierville, TN. Penny can be reached at penny@pennyreed.com or at 1.888.877.5648.

Acknowledgments

I wish to personally thank the following people for their inspiration and support in the development and publication of this book.

To Dr. David Ijams for choosing me to be your office manager and for helping me believe in myself and my dreams.

To Dr. Steve Kail for your mentorship, coaching and partnership, which taught me a great deal about being a coach, running a business and teaching others to have a successful practice.

To Mark LeBlanc, who directed me to turn the seed of an idea into a roadmap for dental business owners. Thank you for being an awesome mentor and friend.

To Henry DeVries, Devin DeVries, Joni McPherson, and the team at Indie Books International. Thank you for your guidance and expertise.

To my team who spent countless hours listening to me talk about this book and pouring over the text for the book. I appreciate your dedication and sharing in the excitement of this project.

To my husband, Rob, whose support and belief in me gave me the confidence to get this message on paper. Thank you for your continuous love and support.

Made in the USA
Columbia, SC
02 October 2022

68303608R00100